# Practical Autonomy
# and Bioethics

# Routledge Annals of Bioethics

EDITED BY MARK J. CHERRY, *St Edwards University, USA*
ANA SMITH ILTIS, *Saint Louis University, USA*

**1. Research Ethics**
Edited by Ana Smith Iltis

**2. Thomistic Principles and Bioethics**
Jason T. Eberl

**3. The Ethics of Genetic Engineering**
Roberta M. Berry

**4. Legal Perspectives in Bioethics**
Edited by Ana S. Iltis, Sandra H.
Johnson, and Barbara A. Hinze

**5. Biomedical Research and Beyond**
Expanding the Ethics of Inquiry
Christopher O. Tollefsen

**6. Practical Autonomy and Bioethics**
James Stacey Taylor

**Previous Titles:**

**Regional Perspectives in Bioethics**
Edited by Mark J. Cherry and
John F. Peppin

**Religious Perspectives on Bioethics**
Edited by Mark J. Cherry, Ana Iltis, and
John F. Peppin

# Practical Autonomy
# and Bioethics

## James Stacey Taylor

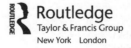

Routledge
Taylor & Francis Group
New York   London

First published 2009
by Routledge
270 Madison Ave, New York, NY 10016

Simultaneously published in the UK
by Routledge
2 Park Square, Milton Park, Abingdon, Oxon OX14 4RN

*Routledge is an imprint of the Taylor & Francis Group, an informa business*

© 2009 Taylor & Francis

Transferred to digital printing 2010

Typeset in Sabon by IBT Global.

*Library of Congress Cataloging-in-Publication Data*
Taylor, James Stacey, 1970–
    Practical autonomy and bioethics / by James Stacey Taylor.
       p. cm. — (Routledge annals of bioethics ; v. 6)
    Includes bibliographical references and index.
1. Autonomy (Psychology)    2. Autonomy (Philosophy)    3. Bioethics.    I. Title.
    BF575.A88T39 2009
    174'.957—dc22
    2009003458

ISBN10: 0-415-99740-2 (hbk)
ISBN10: 0-415-89056-X (pbk)
ISBN10: 0-203-87399-8 (ebk)
ISBN13: 978-0-415-99740-9 (hbk)
ISBN13: 978-0-415-89056-4 (pbk)
ISBN13: 978-0-203-87399-1 (ebk)

*For my parents, Tom and Betty*

# Contents

*Acknowledgments*                                                      ix
*Introduction*                                                         xiii

1   A Theory of Autonomy                                                1

2   The Many Faces of Autonomy?                                        18

3   Identification and Autonomy: A Tale of Two Concepts                37

4   Decisive Identification                                            51

5   Autonomy and Normativity                                           63

6   Autonomy and Choice                                                83

7   Autonomy and Constraint                                            96

8   Autonomy, Privacy, and Patient Confidentiality                    114

9   Autonomy and Informed Consent                                     130

10  The Value of Autonomy in Bioethics                               141

    Conclusion                                                        157

*Notes*                                                               159
*Bibliography*                                                        197
*Index*                                                               207

# Acknowledgments

I first became interested in the nature and value of personal autonomy while working on my MA at St. Andrews University under the tutorship of Professor John Haldane and then Gordon Graham. The interest deepened during my work on my MLitt dissertation at St. Andrews University under the supervision of Sandra Marshall of the University of Stirling, and continued during my MA and PhD work at Bowling Green State University, culminating in my doctoral dissertation on the topic of *Personal Autonomy: Its Philosophical Foundations and Role in Applied Ethics*. Although none of the arguments in those works survived the critical scrutiny that they have subsequently been subjected to (with the exception of some of the ideas concerning the relationship between privacy and autonomy discussed in Chapter 8 of this volume) I thank John Haldane, Gordon Graham, Sandra Marshall and the members of my PhD committee—R. G. Frey, the late James W. Child, Fred D. Miller Jr., and Marina A. L. Oshana—for their support and encouragement of my work. I owe an especially tremendous debt of gratitude to Gordon Graham, who helped me secure a University Scholarship to pursue my MLitt degree at St. Andrews University, and without whose support and encouragement I might not have continued to pursue my philosophical studies.

Although the views in this volume stem from my postgraduate research, it is only since I joined the Department of Philosophy and Religious Studies at The College of New Jersey (TCNJ) that I have been afforded the opportunity to develop them into the form that they now take. As such, I owe a tremendous debt of gratitude to my colleagues at TCNJ— Joanne Cantor, Holly Haynes, Rick Kamber, Pierre LeMorven, Consuelo Preti, Melinda Roberts, John Sisko, and Morton Winston—for providing an academic environment that is both wonderfully collegial and highly conducive to scholarship. I also thank TCNJ for awarding me a three-year Support of Scholarly Activities Award that enabled me to complete this volume, and the staff of TCNJ Library for their sterling works in securing me the materials that I needed.

I am also very grateful for the support that I have received in writing this volume from both the Institute for Humane Studies and the Social

Philosophy & Policy Center at Bowling Green State University. The Institute for Humane Studies not only supported my graduate work on autonomy and bioethics through a series of fellowships but also organized a Current Research Workshop on my work in Stanford, at which my work was subject to rigorous criticism by Michael Bratman, John Christman, Jeremy Shearmur, Yonatan Shemmer, and Mark Reiff, without which this volume would have been much poorer. The Social Philosophy & Policy Center at Bowling Green State University awarded me a Visiting Scholarship for the summer of 2007, during which I wrote Chapters 5, 7, and 10. I thank my research assistants for that summer, Ben Dyer and Richard McNeillie, for their tremendous help, as well as Fred D. Miller Jr., Ellen Frankel Paul, and Jeffrey Paul for providing one of the most conducive places to conduct scholarly research that I have ever known. I also thank Mary Dilsaver, Tammi Sharp, and Terri Weaver of the Social Philosophy & Policy Center, and Joanne Cantor of TCNJ, for the administrative support that they have afforded me. I also (and especially) thank Margy DeLuca of Bowling Green State University for all of the support, encouragement, and administrative help that she has provided, both during my graduate work at Bowling Green, and beyond.

I have discussed various chapters and sections of this volume (and papers that were ancestors of them) at conferences, colloquia, and seminars held at New College Oxford University, University of Leeds, Brown University, Harvard University, University of Southampton, University of Texas at San Antonio, St. Norbert College, Purdue University—Calumet, Boston University, Central Michigan University, University of North Carolina at Chapel Hill, University of Tennessee—Knoxville, East Tennessee State University, Stanford University, University of Boulder—Colorado, University of Florida, The Murphy Institute at Tulane University, The College of New Jersey, Molloy College, University of Virginia, Fordham University, and Bowling Green State University. I thank all who contributed to the discussion on those occasions. I also thank everyone who has given me constructive feedback on drafts of this work, including Michael Almeida, Joel Anderson, Denis Arnold, Nomy Arpaly, Nigel Ashford, Mark Aulisio, Tom L. Beauchamp, Mark Bernstein, Bernard Berofsky, Kimberly Blessing, Mark Brady, Amanda Brand, Michael Bratman, Xunwu Chen, Mark J. Cherry, Damon Chetson, James F. Childress, John Christman, David Copp, Paul Coulam, Stefaan E. Cuypers, Austin Dacey, John Davenport, John Davis, Andy Egan, Laura Waddel Ekstrom, John Martin Fischer, Harry Frankfurt, R. G. Frey, Joshua Gert, Gordon Graham, Jason Grinnell, Camilla Groth, Ishtiyaque Haji, John Haldane, John Heil Jr., John Hernandez, Ben Hippen, John Holder, Robert Hood, Paul M. Hughes, Ana Iltis, Paul Johnson, Rick Kamber, Jason Kawall, William Kline, Robert Kolb, Sigurdur Kristinsson, Hugh LaFollette, Keith Lehrer, Pierre LeMorven, Eric Mack, Thomas May, Rob McDonald, Michael McKenna, Jennifer McKitrick, Fiona McPherson, Al Mele, Fred D. Miller Jr., Jeffrey Moriarty, Paul Naquin, Mike Nichols, Robert Noggle, Marina A. L. Oshana, James

Otteson, Daniel Palmer, Geoffrey Plauche, Consuelo Preti, Francois Raffoul, David Reidy, Mark Reiff, Henry Richardson, Melinda Roberts, John Rowan, Gregory Schrufreider, Jeremy Shearmur, Yonatan Shemmer, David Shoemaker, Mary Sirridge, John Sisko, Rhonda Smith, James Spence, Aaron Spital, Margaret Taylor-Ulizio, Christopher Tollefsen, Paul Tudico, Lars Ursin, Mikhail Valdman, Jukka Varelius, Manuel Vargas, Steven Wall, Gregory Walters, Chad Wilcox, T. M. Wilkinson, Morton Winston, Samuel Zinaich Jr., and many anonymous referees. I especially thank the anonymous referee for Routledge who read an earlier draft of this volume and whose exceptionally insightful and helpful comments pressed me to make it a much stronger work than it would have otherwise been.

I also thank Mark J. Cherry and Ana Iltis for their encouragement during the writing of this volume, especially during its closing stages!

An earlier version of Chapter 8 was published as "Privacy and Autonomy: A Reappraisal," *Southern Journal of Philosophy* 40, no. 4 (2002): 459–473; the material that is reprinted here appears with kind permission of the *Southern Journal of Philosophy*. Sections of Chapter 9 were originally published as "Autonomy and Informed Consent: A Much Misunderstood Relationship," *Journal of Value Inquiry* 38, no. 3 (2004): 383–391; they are reprinted here with kind permission of Springer Science and Business Media.

Finally, I thank my beloved wife, Margaret, and my beloved daughter, Octavia, for their unceasing love and support during both the writing of this volume and the research that went into it, and the dogs, Speckles, Pepper, Sparkles, and the cats, the late Hamish, Nestor (who was almost constantly by my side while I was writing), Lillian, Pia, Peen, the late Case, Little Mum, Dum-Dum, Colours, Button, Frannie, and Evil Mum, for being pets.

# Introduction

It is generally accepted that the value of autonomy is preeminent within contemporary Western bioethics.[1] The conception of autonomy that is at issue here is not, however, that of Kant, on which a person is autonomous only if he conforms his will to the self-imposed dictates of the impersonal moral law. Rather, the conception of autonomy that has come to play a central role in contemporary Western bioethics is that of *personal* autonomy, on which (loosely) a person is autonomous if he guides and directs his decisions and actions in the light of his own desires and values, free from the interference of others.[2] Autonomy has not, however, always enjoyed this exalted position in Western bioethics—or, indeed, in philosophical discussion in general. As Tom L. Beauchamp has noted, there was no indexed mention of "autonomy" in the eight-volume *Encyclopedia of Philosophy* that was published in 1967.[3] And even as recently as 1988 John Christman was able truthfully to write that, outside the Kantian tradition, autonomy "is a comparatively *un*analyzed notion."[4]

Autonomy's meteoric rise to its current status as being of preeminent value in contemporary Western bioethics is no doubt the result of a combination of several factors. As H. Tristram Engelhardt Jr. has argued, the move away from Christian morality as the guiding normative framework within Western ethical discussions had led to an increased pluralism within such debates, which accordingly now lack both "a content-full, generally accepted understanding of the good life and of proper conduct" and "agreement about how one should remedy this difficulty and establish a canonical content-full ethics with its appropriate bioethics."[5] Given this plurality, argues Engelhardt, bioethics has turned away from offering substantive advice and towards the development of a procedural framework for decision-making that is intended to accommodate the fact that cooperating persons might have different value systems.[6] This increasing focus on the development of a procedural framework for bioethical decision-making coincided with a rapid increase in philosophical interest in personal autonomy, an interest that was generated in large part by the publication in 1971 of Harry G. Frankfurt's seminal paper "Freedom of the Will and the Concept of a Person."[7] This combination of the bioethical movement towards a procedural framework for decision-making and the burgeoning philosophical interest in autonomy led naturally to bioethicists coming to focus on respect for autonomy as a way to enable persons with different value systems cooperatively to navigate bioethical issues that affect them. Moreover, as Gerald Dworkin has argued, the importance of autonomy in moral discussion stems also from the plausible view that autonomy must be of fundamental importance for anyone who adheres to a comprehensive moral doctrine. This is because, he argues, such a person must value her autonomy, for it is this that allows her to attempt to live her life in accordance with morality in the first place.[8]

Whatever the reasons for its current status, however, it is undeniable that the value of autonomy is preeminent in contemporary Western bioethics.[9] Given this, it is striking that there has been no concerted effort made by either bioethicists or autonomy theorists to develop and defend an account of personal autonomy that is both theoretically defensible and captures the contours of this concept as it is discussed in contemporary bioethics and contemporary moral philosophy in general. This volume will rectify this lacuna in both the bioethical and action theoretic literatures by developing an account of autonomy that achieves both of these aims. This account of *practical* autonomy—so called because of its explicit genesis as an account of autonomy for discussions of philosophical issues of practical concern, such as the question of the morality of organ sales, or questions concerning the appropriate extent of patient confidentiality—will be both theoretically richer and more defensible than its rivals, as well as being better able to illuminate those debates in both moral philosophy and bioethics in which this concept plays a central role.

In addition to rectifying this lacuna in both the literature on autonomy and the literature on bioethics the discussion of autonomy in this volume will be striking in several other important respects. First, the account of autonomy that will be developed in Chapter 1 will be one that is radically *externalist*, such that a person's autonomy with respect to her decisions and actions will depend in part on the mental states of others. Second, it will be argued that despite the yeoman service that Frankfurt's essay has performed in stimulating philosophical interest in autonomy it has been systematically misunderstood by both autonomy theorists and bioethicists alike. Rather than developing an account of autonomy Frankfurt was, in that essay, developing an account of identification; of what conditions must be met for a person to be said to "identify with" her effective first-order desires, such that when she was moved to act by them she did so freely and of her own free will.[10] As will be argued in Chapter 3, the widespread understanding of Frankfurt's account of *identification* as being an account of autonomy has led to significant confusion in analyzing both concepts. Recognizing and rectifying this will go a long way towards gaining a proper understanding of each of them. Third, the relationships that hold among autonomy, choice, and constraint will be explored, with it being argued that many of the standard views that concern them are mistaken. Contra current received philosophical opinion, it will be argued, respect for a person's autonomy does not generally require that her choices be limited—an argument that has immediate implications for (for example) the debate concerning the morality of current markets in human organs. With this point in hand it will then be argued that autonomy *is* compatible with constraint—and, indeed, a person's exercise of her autonomy *requires* that she be constrained in certain ways, a position that is not incompatible with that concerning autonomy and choice outlined previously. Fourth, revisionary accounts of the relationships that hold between a concern for practical autonomy and concerns with patient privacy and informed consent will be developed. These revisionary accounts of these relationships will lead to the final point of this volume that will be argued for in Chapter 10: that rather than being of intrinsic value, the value of autonomy in bioethics is primarily instrumental.

Having noted the ways in which the account of practical autonomy that will be developed in this volume will enhance the contemporary understanding both of this concept as well as of those debates in contemporary bioethics in which it plays a central role it would be useful to outline how this volume will achieve these ends. In Chapter 1 the connotative contours of the concept of autonomy as these appear in both the autonomy literature and the literature on bioethics will be outlined. With these in hand, the account of practical autonomy that will be the mainstay of the arguments in this volume will be developed and defended. With this account of autonomy in place it will be argued in Chapter 2 that, despite concerns to the contrary, the apparently diverse understandings of autonomy that appear in both the literature on autonomy and the literature on bioethics are not as varied as they might seem. In Chapter 3, it will be argued that autonomy and identification are distinct concepts—a point that will be reinforced in Chapter 4 with the development of a decision-based account of identification. In Chapter 5 it will be argued that, despite appearances, the account of autonomy that was developed in Chapter 1 is a minimally substantive account of autonomy, rather than a content-neutral account. That is, it is one that requires that for a person to be autonomous with respect to her decisions and consequent actions she must endorse certain values. On the face of it, this substantive approach to autonomy might appear to undermine its usefulness as a guiding value for the development of a framework for bioethical decision-making within a pluralistic society. As will be argued in Chapter 5, however, this concern with the value for bioethics of the account of autonomy developed in this volume is misplaced, for not only will the value-commitments that this account will require be minimal but they will be those that any plausible account of autonomy must impose. With this further development and defense of this account of practical autonomy in hand, the ways in which persons' autonomy could be affected both by increasing the numbers of options that are available to them and by subjecting them to constraints will be considered in Chapters 6 and 7. In Chapters 8 and 9 the relationships that hold between concern for the maintenance of patient confidentiality and the securing of patients' informed consent to their treatments will be considered, with revisionary accounts of both being developed. With the discussions of Chapters 6, 8, and 9 in hand, it will be argued in Chapter 10 that autonomy possesses instrumental, rather than intrinsic, value. This volume will conclude with an overview of its main claims.

# 1   A Theory of Autonomy

## INTRODUCTION

It is widely recognized among both autonomy theorists and bioethicists that the term "autonomy" is used in many different ways.[1] This gives rise to what can be called the Gertrude Stein Problem: that when it comes to autonomy, "there is no there there."[2] That is, there seems to be no shared understanding of autonomy that is sufficiently thick to serve as the basis for any analysis of this concept that is widely accepted. This Problem has not gone unrecognized by bioethicists; indeed, three prominent bioethicists (Harry Yeide Jr., Susan J. Dwyer, and, most recently, H. Tristam Engelhardt Jr.) have independently published papers whose titles reflect their concerns with "The Many Faces of Autonomy" in bioethics.[3] This concern on the part of bioethicists to address the Gertrude Stein Problem is understandable, for the prominence of autonomy within bioethics is implicitly based upon the view that the participants in the discussions that draw upon it have a shared understanding of this concept, and that this shared understanding will remain after the concept has been analyzed. If, however, it transpires that there is no shared understanding of autonomy that is widely accepted, then things will look bleak for many discussions within contemporary bioethics. At best, the discussions of the bioethical issues in which autonomy was thought to play a central role will become fractured, with their participants turning only to discuss the issues at hand with others who turn out to share their understanding of autonomy. At worst, it could be that the participants in the bioethical debates in which autonomy plays a central role have simply been talking past each other and turn out not to have any common ground concerning their respective uses of the term "autonomy" from which to continue their discussions.

It is thus important for contemporary bioethics that the Gertrude Stein Problem be addressed. The first possible response to this Problem is to hold that it is illusory: that there is a univocal understanding of autonomy that simply needs to be uncovered.[4] The second response to it—and that which will be pursued in this volume—is more modest. This is to accept that there is no univocal understanding of autonomy, and, from this, develop a "capturing" analysis of autonomy that, while partially stipulative, captures most elements of what most people who use the term philosophically understand by it—and which provides reasons as to why the elements that are not included in it are omitted.

Since the approach to developing an analysis of autonomy that will be pursued here is based on accepting that autonomy is not a univocal concept before embarking upon developing the analysis of autonomy that will be the mainstay of this volume it is necessary to outline the generally accepted connotative contours of this concept as it is used in contemporary philosophical discussion. Outlining these contours will not only provide a basis for the development of a partially stipulative analysis of autonomy, but it could also serve the useful purpose of enabling one to assess just how divergent current understandings of autonomy are. This could then show that the concept of autonomy is not as hydra-headed as it might at first appear, by enabling one to recognize that many of the ways in which "autonomy" is used simply fail to capture the connotative contours of this term, and so are not accounts of autonomy proper. In a related vein, outlining the connotative contours of the concept of autonomy could also enable the proponents of such a capturing analysis of autonomy to claim that it should be accepted as a (or even the) core account of autonomy against which claims about autonomy in those areas of philosophy in which it plays a central role should be assessed. Of course, this latter claim cannot be supported solely by noting that the account of autonomy for which this status is claimed is a capturing account, for this claim might also be made by other, competing, analyses of this concept. One will thus also have to show that competing accounts of autonomy *fail* to be capturing accounts. This additional, negative, claim does not, however, have to made and supported prior to developing a capturing analysis of autonomy, and so it can be left until the next chapter.

It is, then, now time to develop the account of personal autonomy that will be the cornerstone of this volume, and that is intended to help illuminate those discussions in moral philosophy in general, and bioethics in particular, in which this concept plays a central role.

## THE CONNOTATIVE CONTOURS OF AUTONOMY

As noted previously, prior to developing an analysis of autonomy it is sensible to outline the connotative contours of this concept. Turning first to the positive aspects of autonomy, it is generally accepted that autonomy is a property of persons, rather than of nonpersons, such as very small children, wantons, or animals.[5] Persons are held to be able to direct themselves in ways that are not open to other agents. They are able to reflect on their inclinations, desires, and values to determine if they wish to be moved by them or not. As such, autonomy is primarily a property of persons with respect to their local attributes, such as their choices, their effective first-order desires, their preferences, and their actions.[6] Thus, insofar as persons are held to be autonomous simpliciter, such a global attribution of autonomy will be based upon the number and importance of their local features with respect to which they possess it. Given this, it is clear that persons can enjoy autonomy to differing degrees, for they could enjoy autonomy both with respect to a greater or lesser number of their local attributes and also could possess or lack autonomy with respect to those attributes that are of more or less importance to them.[7] Finally, it is generally accepted that the actions of autonomous persons are not subject to the direction of others, as a slave's actions are subject to the directions of his master, or a soldier's are subject to the directions of his officers.[8]

Turning now to the negative aspects of autonomy, that is, to those phenomena that are generally held to compromise a person's autonomy with respect to his decisions, or his effective first-order desires, or his actions, it is generally accepted that a person who is coerced into performing an action suffers from a diminution in his autonomy with respect to it.[9] For example, a person who is coerced by a family member into selling a kidney thereby suffers from a diminution in her autonomy with respect to that sale. Similarly, a person is generally held to suffer from a diminution in his autonomy with respect to his decisions, and the desires and actions that flow from them, if he was deceived or unknowingly manipulated into making them. If, for example, a physician withholds information about the side effects of a drug to encourage his patient to take it, the patient will suffer from a diminution in his autonomy with respect to his taking of the drug. It is also widely believed that a person who is subject to brainwashing, beset by unwanted addictions or mired in poverty, would suffer from compromised autonomy. It is also generally believed that a person who lacks independence of mind and who blindly follows the lead of others will be less likely to possess autonomy. Similarly, persons who lack minimal rationality, or who suffer from neuroses, compulsions, or ambivalence about the choices that they make, are held to enjoy autonomy only to a low degree with respect to them, if they even possess it at all.[10] Thus, Paul M. Hughes argues, since persons would typically be ambivalent about the sale of a bodily organ, the typical organ vendor would suffer from compromised autonomy with respect to any such sales that she makes.[11]

## MANIPULATION, DECEPTION, AND PERSONAL AUTONOMY

These connotative contours of the concept of autonomy can now be used as a template from which a capturing analysis of this concept can be developed. This analysis will not only capture the commonly accepted connotative contours of autonomy but, insofar as it does not, it can be used to explain why those that it *fails* to capture are the results of misguided intuitions about autonomy. The analysis of autonomy that will be developed here will also be an account of *practical* autonomy. That is, it will be judgmentally relevant to those debates in moral philosophy in general, and bioethics in particular, in which the concept of personal autonomy plays a central role.

It is sensible to begin developing this account of practical autonomy by referring to the ways in which a person's autonomy can be compromised. As noted before, it is generally accepted that when a person is manipulated into performing an action he suffers from a diminution in his autonomy with respect to that action.[12] To see this, consider the example of Othello and Iago from Shakespeare's *Othello*.[13] *Othello* begins with an argument between Iago and Roderigo that was started as a result of Roderigo learning that despite his employment of Iago to help further his suit to Desdemona, Desdemona has just married Othello, the general that Iago serves as an ensign. Iago already dislikes Othello because he has passed him over for promotion to lieutenant in favor of the less experienced Cassio, and so he determines to bring about the ruin of both Cassio and Othello. Naturally, Roderigo is concerned to aid in the ruin of Othello, and when Iago convinces him that Desdemona will seek satisfaction with Cassio once she becomes tired of Othello he is keen to aid in the ruin of this apparent rival also. Iago arranges for it to appear to Othello that Cassio started a fight with Roderigo which leads to his demotion. He then convinces Cassio that the best way to get back into Othello's good graces is to use Desdemona as an intermediary, planning to frame them as lovers. Iago achieves his latter goal through a serious of insinuations, manipulating Othello into believing that Cassio and Desdemona are having an affair. Iago acquires a handkerchief that Othello gave to Desdemona after Othello dropped it and plants it in Cassio's room. Cassio, wondering where it came from, asks Bianca, a prostitute, to copy its embroidery for him. Iago then arranges for Othello to overhear Bianca challenge Cassio for asking her to copy the embroidery from a love token given to him by another woman. Othello becomes convinced of the affair and is thereby led to smother Desdemona.

Since Othello was manipulated by Iago into smothering Desdemona, he lacked autonomy with respect to his decision to do this, for it was not he, but Iago, who was the font of this decision. It was not Othello, but Iago, who originally decided to cause Desdemona's death; Othello was merely the instrument through which he brought this about.[14] This last point is important, for it highlights the way in which Iago's control over Othello through his control over the information that Othello had access to undermined Othello's autonomy with respect to his decisions (and hence his consequent effective first-order desires and actions). To see this clearly, consider a similar example developed by Alfred Mele. In Mele's example an ideally self-controlled king, King George, rules his kingdom based on information supplied by his staff, who systematically deceive him to ensure that the better he deliberates the worse his kingdom becomes according to his own values and principles. King George, Mele writes, is because of this "heteronomous in a significant sphere of his life," for he is "information-ally cut off from ruling autonomously."[15] Mele's example of King George is thus similar to the example of Iago and Othello.[16] However, the reason Mele believes that King George's informational deprivation precluded him from being autonomous with respect to his ruling of his kingdom is that it precluded him from *successfully* achieving his ends.[17] Given this, accord-ing to Mele, King George would suffer from a similar lack of autonomy with respect to his rule were his misinformation to arise from some nonin-tentional source.[18] But Mele is mistaken here. To see this, consider a revi-sion of the example of Iago and Othello.[19] In this revised example (written, perhaps, by a Scottish Shakespeare), the physical actions of McIago and McOthello are precisely the same as those that occurred between Iago and Othello in the original English play—and they bring about the same lethal results for McDesdemona. However, there is one crucial difference. In this fictitious Scottish version of *Othello* McIago lacked all guile and cunning, and merely reported to McOthello the facts as he saw them. Unlike Iago, then, McIago did not intend to direct McOthello's decisions or actions at all. As such, in *McOthello* McOthello was, unlike Othello, directing him-self, rather than being under the direction of another. It was he, and not McIago, who was the font of the decision to kill McDesdemona. McIago was merely providing him with the information upon which he acted and was not directing his decisions and actions at all. Thus, whereas in *Othello* Iago *intended* to direct Othello's decisions and actions and, in successfully getting Othello to decide and act as he wanted successfully exercised con-trol over him, in *McOthello* McIago exercised no such control over McO-thello, since it was not he, but McOthello, who decided what decisions and what actions McOthello should make. As such, then, while Othello suf-fered from a diminution in his autonomy with respect to his decisions and actions insofar as they were under the control of Iago, McOthello suffered from no such diminution in his autonomy.[20] Mele is thus mistaken to hold that King George would have suffered from a diminution in his autonomy with respect to his decisions and actions had the informational encapsu-lation that precluded him from achieving his ends in ruling his kingdom arisen from a nonintentional source. This is because the crucial differ-ence between Othello, who suffered from a diminution in his autonomy with respect to his decisions and actions, and McOthello, who did not, is that the former—and not the latter—was subject to the control of another agent, the exercise of which required that the agent in question *intended* to control his decisions and actions. Absent such intentional control, then, King George would have been directing his own decisions and actions, and so he could have been fully autonomous with respect to them, no matter how unsuccessful his exercise of his autonomy might have been in achiev-ing his ends.[21]

To underscore this point, consider the case of Martin Frobisher, who in 1576 explored Baffin Island and returned to England with a quantity of minerals that he thought was gold but which turned out to be iron pyrites. Undaunted by this failure, Frobisher returned to Canada in 1577, and again in 1578; both times his ships returned to England loaded with worthless iron pyrites. Like Mele's King George, Frobisher's ignorance (in his case, of geology) precluded him from successfully achieving his ends, for it led him to continue to return to an area where gold was unavailable. However, that Frobisher's ignorance led to his being informationally cut off from achieving his ends does not show that he lacked autonomy with respect to his decisions to return to Canada and bring back ore to England and the consequent actions that he performed to achieve these ends. Frobisher's decisions and actions were still under his control—and not that of another person. It was still he, and not someone else, who was deciding what decisions he would make and what actions he would perform; he was thus autonomous, self-directed, with respect to them. Yet although Frobisher was autonomous with respect to both his decisions and the actions that flowed from them, his geological ignorance precluded him from exercising his autonomy in a way that would achieve his goals. As such, then, rather than undermining his autonomy *per se* Frobisher's informational removal from being able to achieve his ends compromised only the *instrumental value* of his autonomy to him. Rather than holding that King George's autonomy would be undermined were his informational encapsulation to arise from a nonintentional source, then, Mele should instead have held that even though in such a case King George might still have been fully autonomous with respect to his decisions and his actions, his autonomy would have had little to no instrumental value for him. This claim captures the view that something has gone awry with respect to King George's autonomy when he is exercising it under adverse epistemic conditions and yet avoids committing Mele to holding that King George suffered from a diminution in his autonomy even though it was still he—and not someone else—who was directing the making of his decisions and the performance of his actions.

## A THEORY OF PRACTICAL AUTONOMY

### The Threshold Condition

From the examples of King George and Othello it is clear that if a person's decisions are subject to the control of another person as a result of her controlling the information that he is basing them on, he will suffer from a diminution in his autonomy with respect to them. From this, the first condition for a person to be autonomous with respect to his decisions (the "threshold condition," since it marks the threshold for a person to be autonomous with respect to her decisions simpliciter) can be developed:

Threshold Condition: It is necessary for a person to be autonomous with respect to a decision that she makes that (i) the information on which she based the decision has not been affected by another agent with the end of leading her to make a particular decision, or a decision from a particular class of decisions.

As it stands, however, this condition is too restrictive, for it would preclude a person who makes a decision on the basis of another person's advice from being autonomous with respect to it. And this is clearly mistaken, for were McOthello merely to seek the (unmanipulative) advice of McIago his decisions would still be under his control, for he could accept or reject it as he saw fit. This Threshold Condition, then, should be supplemented with a caveat:

(ii) if the information on which a person makes her decision has been affected by another agent with the end of leading her to make a particular decision, or a decision from a particular class of decisions, she is aware of the way in which it has been so affected.[22]

Yet even with this caveat in place the Threshold Condition is still too restrictive. This is because a person could make decisions that are based, in part, upon information that has been affected by another agent with the end of leading her to make a particular choice, or a choice from a particular class of choices, *without* making the decision that the other agent in question was intended her to make. For example, on coming to believe that Desdemona was being unfaithful to him, instead of smothering her Othello might have sought out marriage counseling. In this "New Man" version of Othello, it would still be Othello, and not Iago, who would be in control of his decisions and, hence, his actions, and so he would be autonomous with respect to them. To accommodate this, the Threshold Condition needs a further supplement:

(iii) if the information on which a person bases her decision has been affected by another agent with the end of leading her to make a particular decision, or a decision from a particular class of decisions, and if she is not aware of the way in which the information on which she is basing her decision has been so affected, then she did not make the decision that the agent who was affecting the information she had access to with the intent of leading her to make a particular decision intended her to make.[23]

## The Degree Condition

The Threshold Condition provides a set of requirements that are necessary for a person to be autonomous with respect to her decisions. As it stands, however, it does not provide a set of sufficient conditions for persons to be autonomous with respect to their decisions. It is possible, for example, that certain clearly nonautonomous wanton agents, such as very small children, could meet the Threshold Condition for autonomy. Moreover, the Threshold Condition fails to capture the fact that persons can be more or less autonomous with respect to their decisions.[24] A person who makes an uncharacteristically snap decision on the spur of the moment would not, for example, be as autonomous with respect to it as he would be with respect to a decision that he made with his characteristic care. Such a person would not be fully self-directed with respect to how he made his decision, for insofar as the decision-making procedure that he used was not one that he endorsed he would not be fully directing himself in accord with his own desires and values since his decision-making procedure itself would fail to reflect them. The cases of the nonautonomous wanton and the snap decision maker thus show that to be autonomous with respect to his decisions a person must have reflected upon the decision-making procedures that they are produced by, and that he accepts the procedures that he uses as his own. The degree to which a person is autonomous with respect to his decisions will thus be determined in part by the degree to which they are the result of a decision-making procedure that he is satisfied with as being his, where such satisfaction consists solely in his being unmoved to alter it after he has become aware of how he makes his decisions.[25] More formally:

> Degree Condition: The maximum degree to which a person will be au-
> tonomous with respect to a decision that she makes will be determined
> by the degree to which it is the result of a decision-making procedure
> that she is satisfied with as being her decision-making procedure for
> making the type of the decision that is in question; to the degree that
> the genesis of her decision departs from this she will suffer from a dimi-
> nution on her autonomy with respect to the decision in question.

Four points are worth making with respect to the Degree Condition. First, on the notion of satisfaction that is used here a person will be satisfied with a decision-making procedure if she believes that she has sufficient reason to continue using it. As such, then, a person need not believe that the decision-making procedure that she is using is that which is optimal for her, although she must believe that it will result in decisions that are normative for her; that is, she must believe that she has reason to act on the decisions that she makes through using it.[26] Second, it is possible that a person might be satisfied with more than one decision-making procedure. For example, a man might be careful and meticulous in making decisions about his medical treatments yet impetuous and spontaneous in making decisions in his personal life—and be satisfied with both of these decision-making procedures in their respective realms. Following from this second point, it must be stressed that this focus upon a person's decision-making procedure does not accord any special significance to the sort of intellectual, rationalistic deliberations favored by (for example) academic philosophers.[27] A person's decision-making procedure could be rash, impetuous, or spontaneous—all that matters is that it is one that she is satisfied with in the sense outlined previously.[28] Finally, in requiring that the degree to which a person is autonomous with respect to her decisions be partially determined by the degree to which they originate from a decision-making procedure that she is satisfied with the Degree Condition serves to differentiate autonomous from nonautonomous agents. In requiring that to be autonomous with respect to her decisions an agent must be aware of her decision-making procedure the Degree Condition imposes upon agents a requirement that they must be reflexively self-aware to be autonomous with respect to their decisions. As such, agents such as animals, very small children, or even utterly unreflective adult humans will lack autonomy with respect to their decisions on this analysis of autonomy—ascriptions of heteronomy that fit with widely held intuitions concerning the limits of the range of autonomous agents. However, although the Degree Condition precludes such agents from being autonomous with respect to their decisions, it does not preclude *all* wantons from being autonomous.

To see this, consider Captain Grimes, from Evelyn Waugh's novel *Decline and Fall*. Grimes believes that one will avoid long-term unhappiness provided that one "does just exactly what one wants to and when one wants to."[29] Grimes, then, is what Frankfurt termed a "rational wanton."[30] He "is not concerned with the desirability of his desires themselves. He ignores the question of what his will is to be. . ." and he "does not care which of his inclinations is the strongest." However, he can deliberate "upon the suitability of his desires to one course of action or another," and he deliberates "concerning how to do what he wants to do."[31] Yet Grimes's being "singularly in harmony with the primitive promptings of humanity" and his consequent indifference towards which of his desires leads him to act does not preclude him from deliberately directing himself in light of them. For example, having a strong desire to retain his undemanding job at a "pretty bad" public school in Wales and recognizing that he is likely to "land in the soup again" Grimes secretly became engaged to be married to Flossie, one of the daughters of the school's headmaster, with the sole purpose of revealing this as his "last card" should he need to do so to keep his job.[32] Despite this planning to satisfy his desires, however, Grimes never questions their desirability—that he likes his job and that he wants to retain it in the easiest way possible, even though this involves using Flossie as a mere means, is sufficient for him to act upon them. Grimes, then, is a wanton—but a wanton who could satisfy the conditions outlined previously for him to be autonomous with respect to his decisions. Grimes's decision to marry Flossie, for example, was made without the information on which he made it being affected by another person with the end of leading him to make a certain decision, or a decision from a certain class of decisions. It thus satisfies the Threshold Condition. Moreover, it was a decision that was the result of a decision-making procedure that Grimes is satisfied with for making such decisions. Grimes's decision to marry Flossie thus satisfies the Degree Condition—and to a high degree. Grimes, then, is a wanton who is (at least sometimes) autonomous with respect to his decisions.

This claim might strike some persons as being counterintuitive. After all, to be a wanton is often taken to be synonymous with being a nonautonomous agent.[33] On reflection, however, it is clear that the wantonness of a person such as Grimes with respect to his desires is no bar to his being autonomous with respect to his decisions. Grimes makes plans to satisfy his desires, and puts them into action. He is aware of the decision-making procedures that he engages in to do so, and he is satisfied with them in that he is not moved to alter them once he becomes aware of them. Given this, it is not unintuitive to hold that Grimes could be fully self-directed, fully autonomous, with respect to his decisions. One might, though, simply hold that *by definition* wantons cannot be autonomous. There are two reasons why one might accept such a stipulation. The first is that in "Freedom of the Will and the Concept of a Person" Frankfurt used the example of a wanton to illustrate the difference between agents who could be said to identify with their desires (non-wantons) and agents who could not (wantons).[34] However, as will be argued in Chapter 3, Frankfurt's account of what it is for a person to identify with her effective first-order desires is not an account of what it is for a person to be autonomous with respect to them, but an account of what it is for a person to act freely and of her own free will. As such, even if one accepts Frankfurt's taxonomy of which agents act freely and of their own free will and which do not, that Frankfurt holds that a wanton is a paradigmatic example of an agent who does not act freely and of her own free will is orthogonal to the question of whether she is autonomous with respect to her decisions.[35] Alternatively, one might think that a wanton would be precluded from being autonomous with respect to his decisions because he had not endorsed the desires and values on which he was making them. As such, one might argue, agents such as Grimes lack autonomy with respect to their decisions because the desires and values on which they base them are in some sense not fully their own. This requirement that a person must endorse all of her desires and values to be autonomous with respect to those of her decisions that are based on them will be discussed more fully in Chapter 7. However, it can be noted here that this requirement is exceptionally stringent and would result in few, if any, persons being autonomous with respect to their decisions—an outcome that conflicts with the widely held intuition that most persons are autonomous to some degree with respect to most of their decisions. Furthermore, the imposition of such a Requirement of Universal Endorsement would hold only highly reflective and deliberative persons to be autonomous. As will be argued next, this reflects an indefensible and parochial commitment to the value of deliberative reflection over other values, such as spontaneity—and this commitment is by no means part of the concept of personal autonomy.[36]

## The Tracing Condition

One final refinement needs to be added to this account of practical autonomy. It might be that a person decides that although he is satisfied with the decision-making procedures that he is currently using to make his decisions he would like to try something new, to see whether this might improve his ability to satisfy his desires. The first time (perhaps, the first few times) that he uses his new decision-making procedure, however, such a person will not be satisfied with it in the sense outlined above. It will, in effect, be on probation pending its results, and so the person who is using it will be withholding his judgment as to whether he is unmoved to alter it or not. Given the Degree Condition, then, such a person, then, would (on the analysis of autonomy developed so far) be considered to suffer from a diminution in his autonomy with respect to the decisions that he makes using such a probationary decision-making procedure, for it would depart from the decision-making procedures that he is satisfied with as being his. But this is mistaken, for insofar as the person in question chose to experiment with a different decision-making procedure, chose the procedure himself using a decision-making procedure that he was satisfied with, and made his own decisions based on the new procedure that he chose to use, he would be just as self-directed, just as autonomous, as he would have been had he made his decisions based on those procedures that he was already satisfied with. To accommodate this, then, a final condition must be added to this account of autonomy:

> Tracing Condition: If a person decides to use a different decision-making procedure than that which she is satisfied with as being her own, then the maximal degree to which she is autonomous with respect to the decisions that she makes using it will be determined by the degree to which she was autonomous with respect to the decision-making procedure that she used to make the choice to use an alternative decision-making procedure. Her degree of autonomy with respect to the decisions that she makes will then be determined by how closely her actual decision-making procedure that leads to them is in accord with the decision-making procedure that she decided to adopt in making them.

## CLARIFYING AND ELABORATING THIS ACCOUNT OF PRACTICAL AUTONOMY

With this account of practical autonomy in place, it is time to clarify and elaborate it.

### The Scope of Autonomy

On this account of autonomy a person can not only be autonomous with respect to her decisions, but also with respect to her other mental states as well as to her actions, with her autonomy with respect to each of them being accounted for by their relationship to decisions that she was autonomous with respect to. For example, if a person was autonomous with respect to her decision to satisfy one of her preexisting desires (such as her decision to undergo cosmetic surgery) then she would be autonomous to the same degree with respect to that desire when it moved her to act. Similarly, insofar as she was autonomous with respect to the first-order desire that moved her to act then she would be *prima facie* autonomous with respect to the action that it moved her to perform.[37] It is important to note that on this account of autonomy a person is not necessarily alienated from her desires (or the actions that they led her to perform) if she is not autonomous with respect to them. A person might, for example, fail to be aware of one of her decision-making procedures, make a decision on the basis of it, and act to satisfy the desire that she had thus decided to satisfy. Since this person was not aware of the decision-making procedure that she used to decide to satisfy the desire in question, and thus could not be satisfied with it, she would fail to meet the Degree Condition to be autonomous with respect to either the decision or the desire in question. However, that this is so does not mean that she was therefore *alienated* from them, for they might still be *authentically* hers, either qua person or qua agent. To see this, consider the case of a small child, whose decisions, desires, and actions authentically reflect her motivational set. Despite this, the child is too young to be reflexively aware of how she makes decisions, and so fails to be satisfied with them in the way required for her to be autonomous with respect to them. However, since they directly flow from her motivational set she is not alienated from them. As such, on the account of autonomy developed here there is a tripartite taxonomy of effective first-order desires: those that an agent is autonomous with respect to, those that are authentically hers, but which she is heteronomous with respect to, and those that she is alienated from.[38] Noting that it is possible for a person to be heteronomous with respect to her effective first-order desires and yet not alienated from them is important, for it shows that accounts of autonomy that offer merely a negative analysis of the concept as nonalienation will be inaccurate as they are based upon an impoverished taxonomy of desires.[39] For example, consider in this regard John Christman's account of autonomy, on which a person will be autonomous with respect to a desire, D, if she does not, or would not, disown it after reflecting upon the process by which she came to have it.[40] For Christman, an agent, P, is autonomous with respect to her desires (or other pro-attitudes) at a time, t, if-

i. P did not resist the development of D (prior to t) when attending to this process of development, or P would not have resisted that development had P attended to the process;

ii. The lack of resistance to the development of D (prior to t) did not take place (or would not have) under the influence of factors that inhibit self-reflection;

iii. The reflection involved in condition I is (minimally) rational and involves no self-deception;[41] and

iv. The agent is minimally rational with respect to D at t (where minimal rationality demands that an agent experience no manifest conflicts of desires or beliefs that significantly affect the agent's behavior and that are not subsumed under some otherwise rational plan of action).[42]

Yet given this account of what it is for an agent to be autonomous with respect to a desire D at time t Christman has no means of distinguishing between desires possessed by nonautonomous agents (such as, for example, small children) who are authentically their own, and desires that agents are autonomous with respect to.[43] An agent might, for example, possess a desire that she is not "actively derisive of," and which she does not "want to reject and resist," but which nonetheless she is not autonomous with respect to for she has never reflected upon the decision-making procedure that led her to possess it, and so although she is not alienated from it, it is hers only in the same way as a child's authentic desires are hers.[44]

## A Historical Account

The account of practical autonomy that has been developed previously is a historical account of autonomy. That is, it is an account of autonomy on which a person's autonomy with respect to his decisions (desires, and actions) is partially determined by the process by which he came to make (satisfy, or perform) them. If, for example, a person is manipulated into making a decision, as Othello was by Iago, he would not be autonomous with respect to it. Like other historical accounts of autonomy, then, the account developed previously is not vulnerable to the Problem of Manipulation that besets desire-based ahistorical accounts of autonomy on which a person is autonomous with respect to some pro-attitude if it stands in certain structural relationships to her other mental states.[45] As the account of autonomy developed previously requires that a person *decide* to satisfy a desire for him to be autonomous with respect to it, and for the decision-making procedure that he use to do so be one that he is satisfied with, it is immune to the Problem of Manipulation since persons cannot have decisions inculcated into them; they must *make* them.

One might, however, object that persons do not necessarily make decisions but that they could be passive with respect to them, just as they could be with desires. Thus, such a person might claim, since persons can be passive with respect to their decisions, just as a person might have a desire inculcated into her, so too might she have a decision inculcated into her— and so that the previous historical account of autonomy is a decision-based account is no bar to its being subject to the Problem of Manipulation. Support for this objection to the prior account of autonomy can be drawn from an example developed by J. David Velleman, in which

I have a long-anticipated meeting with an old friend for the purpose of resolving some minor difference, but. . . as we talk his offhand comments provoke me to raise my voice in progressively sharper replies, until we part in anger. Later reflection leads me to realize that accumulated grievances had crystallized in my mind, during the weeks before our meeting, into a resolution to sever our friendship over the matter in hand, and that this resolution is what gave the hurtful edge to my remarks. In short, I may conclude that desires of mine caused the decision, which in turn caused the corresponding behavior; and I may acknowledge that these mental states were thereby exerting their normal motivational force. . . But do I necessarily think that I made the decision or that I executed it? Surely, I can believe that the decision. . . was. . . induced in me but not formed by me. . . Indeed, viewing the decision as directly motivated by my desires, and my behavior as directly governed by the decision, is precisely what leads to the thought that as my words became more shrill, it was my resentment speaking, not I.[46]

In this example Velleman claims that he was not active with respect to his decision; he was not autonomous with respect to it because it just came over him, as a wave of resentment might break over someone in the midst of a heated conversation. Yet although Nomy Arpaly claims that Velleman's example is "extremely lifelike" it is not obvious that Velleman's assertion that in this case a *decision* was (passively) caused that led to his behavior is correct.[47] There is nothing in Velleman's example that commits one to accepting that the severing of his friendship was brought about by a decision to do so. Indeed, a more natural understanding of the situation that Velleman outlines is that he possessed a strong and unacknowledged desire to sever the friendship, that this desire led him to act as he did, and that he came to recognize this when he subsequently reflected on what happened. But this understanding of the situation not only obviates the need to claim that the severing of the friendship was brought about by a decision that he was somehow passive with respect to but it places Velleman's motivational passivity with respect to the severing firmly at the doorstep of his desire to do so—and the possible passivity of a person with respect to his effective desires is acknowledged by all. Since Velleman's behavior can be fully explained without introducing a reference to a decision, the application of Occam's Razor would suggest that none be introduced. Moreover, it is not clear what Velleman means when he writes that "Surely, I can believe that the decision. . .was induced in me but not formed by me. . ." It appears that he is claiming that his decision was made for him, rather as he was standing apart from his deliberative process, with his mental states taking on a life of their own. But decisions simply do not creep up on people and materialize before them as they look on passively; they must be made. This is simply part of the nature of a decision. Despite Velleman's assertion to the contrary, then, persons are necessarily active with respect to their decisions, rather than passive in the way that he suggests.

With these points in hand a further elaboration of this model of autonomy is in order. It is usually believed that a person who is beset by an unwanted addiction suffers from a diminution in his autonomy to the extent that he succumbs to his craving.[48] But, if the account of autonomy that has been developed previously is correct, this need not be the case. Consider an unwilling addict who is periodically beset by a craving for nicotine and who suffers greatly until he gives in to it and smokes a cigarette. Such an addict is not simply overwhelmed by his desire for nicotine. Rather, he deliberates as to whether or not he will give in to his craving—and, if so, when he will do so. Even an unwilling addict, then, will decide whether or not to take the drug to which he is addicted, and when he will do this. Thus, if such an addict decides when to take the drug to which he is addicted in accordance with a decision-making procedure that he is satisfied with, he will be autonomous with respect to his taking of the drug.[49] One might think that this serves as a counterexample to the account of autonomy developed above. But this is not so. Such an unwilling addict would, no doubt, take the drug to which he is addicted to avoid the pain that he would otherwise experience were he to continue to resist his craving. Given this, he is like any other agent who finds himself in a situation in which he is faced with a series of options that are unpalatable to him.[50] The mere unpalatability of an agent's option set to him, however, tells us nothing about his ability to make decisions to direct himself through it. It merely tells us that no matter how relatively successful the agent might be at such self-direction it will bring him a low degree of well-being. The unpalatability of the option set faced by the unwilling addict, then, tells us nothing about whether he could be autonomous with respect to the decisions that he makes concerning his addiction but only that his exercise of his autonomy in this situation is likely to be of only low instrumental value to him. The intuition that an unwilling addict somehow suffers from compromised autonomy, then, can be accommodated not at the descriptive level (i.e., he is not less autonomous as a result of his addiction) but at a normative level (i.e., his autonomy is less instrumentally valuable to him).[51]

## A Radically Externalist Account of a Political Concept

In addition to being a decision-based historical account, this account of autonomy is also an *externalist* account. That is to say, on this account of autonomy the issue of whether a person is autonomous with respect to a decision (desire, or action) cannot be determined simply by reference to factors that are internal to her (i.e., her mental states), but must also make reference to her interactions with other people. Moreover, as the previous discussion of *Othello* and the fictitious *McOthello* shows, the question of whether a person was autonomous with respect to a decision cannot be decided merely by observing her interactions with other people, for it will also crucially depend on their mental states. Thus, P's failure to be autonomous with respect to (some of) his decisions could be the result of another person Q's having certain mental states, for P would have been autonomous with respect to the decisions in question were Q to have acted in precisely the same way and had precisely the same effects on P but with different motivations. To put it crudely, but accurately, then, on this account of autonomy the question of whether *I* am autonomous with respect to my decisions (choices, or actions) will depend, in part, on *your* mental states. This point should also lead one to recognize that autonomy is an essentially *political* concept. That is, the concept of autonomy is one where the question of its attribution (e.g., questions concerning whether or not a given person is autonomous with respect to a given decision) will necessarily have to refer to questions concerning the presence or absence of interpersonal influence, whether this influence is conducted by force or without it. This is not to claim, of course, that a person who is isolated from others (such as Robinson Crusoe before the appearance of Friday) and who is thus free from their influence cannot be autonomous with respect to his decisions (or desires, or actions, and so on). But it is to claim that if a person is located in a setting in which his decisions could be subject to the influence of others that the question of whether they are or not (and, if so, in what way) is one that must be addressed prior to attributing autonomy to him with respect to them. Of course, given both the radical externalism of practical autonomy and its consequent political nature there will be significant epistemological problems associated with correctly ascribing autonomy to persons with respect to their decisions (and desires, and actions, and so on) in all cases. This, though, is neither a bar to this account of autonomy being correct (for epistemological questions are distinct from ontological ones), and nor (and more importantly for this account of autonomy as an account of *practical* autonomy) is it a bar to the use of this concept within the context of applied ethics. This is because since persons are not, like Othello, typically unwittingly subject to the control of others it is fair to adopt as the default position the view that unless there is reason to believe otherwise it should not be assumed that persons' autonomy with respect to their decisions (desires, actions, and so on) is compromised through the illegitimate influence of others. Furthermore, given that persons often recognize when they are in situations in which they might be subject to manipulation by others (e.g., when dealing with salesmen, politicians, or even when on a first date), even in potentially manipulative situations part (ii) of the Threshold Condition will often be met. Thus, situations in which persons are unwittingly subject to manipulation are likely to be few and far between. That the application of this account of practical autonomy will be subject to epistemological difficulties that will lead to autonomy being occasionally incorrectly ascribed to (or withheld from) some persons with respect to their decisions (or desires, or actions, and so on) is hence no bar to its correct ascription in the vast majority of cases. Finally, recognizing that autonomy is a radically externalist political concept will lead to questions being raised about how it is to be valued—questions that will be comprehensively addressed in Chapter 10.

## CONCLUSION

The account of practical autonomy that has been developed in this chapter is a decision-based, historical, externalist, and political account. It has several clear advantages as an account of personal autonomy, not the least of which is the fact that it manages to capture the connotative contours of this concept as these were outlined at the start of this chapter. Moreover, as will be discussed later in this volume, the account of autonomy developed here will also be able to be used to explain the relationship between personal autonomy and the availability of choice, the relationship between autonomy and informed consent, and why it is that violating a person's privacy will (typically) compromise her autonomy. As such, it will be an account of autonomy that is exceptionally well placed to serve as the canonical account of this concept as it is used in contemporary bioethics. Yes, despite these advantages of this account of autonomy it still needs to be clarified and defended. In particular, and insofar as it is a value-neutral account of autonomy (that is, an account of autonomy on which a person need not endorse any substantive value-commitments to be autonomous), it must be defended against charges that only substantive accounts of autonomy are tenable, while the scope of deliberation that agents are expected to engage in to be autonomous needs to be clarified. These issues will be addressed in Chapters 5 and 7. It should also be defended against the suspicion that this new account of autonomy is simply another addition to the wide range of accounts of autonomy that already exist; a charge that will be addressed in the next chapter. And, in a similar vein, with this account of autonomy in hand one of the most serious methodological and substantive problems that besets all who work with the concept of autonomy can now be addressed in Chapter 3: the conflation of the concept of autonomy with that of identification.

# 2 The Many Faces of Autonomy?

## INTRODUCTION

It was noted in Chapter 1 that discussions of autonomy in bioethics are beset by the Gertrude Stein Problem: that there is no shared understanding of autonomy that is sufficiently thick to serve as the basis for any analysis of this concept that is widely accepted. It was also noted there that, despite this, it is still possible to develop a capturing account of autonomy that, while partially stipulative, both captures most of the connotative contours of this concept as it is used in contemporary philosophical discussion and is able to explain why those that it does not capture should be excluded as being part of the understanding of autonomy proper. This capturing account of autonomy was the account of practical autonomy that was developed in the last Chapter. It was also noted in Chapter 1 that explicitly outlining the connotative contours of the contemporary philosophical conception of autonomy will enable one to assess just how divergent current understandings of autonomy are. This assessment, it was noted, could serve two useful purposes. First, it could, perhaps, show that the philosophical understanding of autonomy is not as multifaceted as it might at first appear—that this is simply an illusion generated by the widespread usage of this concept in ways that do not track its generally accepted connotations.[1] Second, if this is so, then this assessment would support a claim made on behalf of a capturing account of autonomy to be considered to be a (if not *the*) core account of autonomy against which claims about autonomy in discussions of political philosophy, moral philosophy, and both applied ethics in general, and bioethics in particular, should be assessed.

This chapter will thus address the Gertrude Stein Problem by assessing how well current uses of the term "autonomy" capture the connotative contours of this concept as it is used in contemporary philosophical discussion. Drawing on the connotative contours of the concept of autonomy as these were outlined in Chapter 1 it will be argued that autonomy is not such a hydra-headed concept as it might at first seem. This is because many of what are held to be accounts of autonomy fail as such in one of two ways: they fail to capture one or more (or even all) of the connotative contours of this concept without their proponents being able to provide a principled reason for this omission, or they only capture one of these contours, and so, insofar as they can be subsumed into another account of autonomy, lose their status as independent analyses of this concept.[2] And this is good news for the account of practical autonomy that was developed in Chapter 1, for it supports its claim to be a (if not *the*) core account of autonomy for use in contemporary moral and social philosophy—and especially those contemporary discussions of bioethics in which the concept of autonomy plays a central role.

## VARIETIES OF AUTONOMY?

Having outlined the generally accepted contours of the concept of autonomy in the previous chapter it is time to consider several accounts of autonomy to assess whether they capture them. That autonomy appears to be a hydra-headed concept that has been recognized by the autonomy theorists Joel Feinberg, Gerald Dworkin, Manuel Vargas, and Nomy Arpaly (among others), as well as, as noted in the previous chapter, by many of those who work with this concept in bioethics. Feinberg holds that "the word 'autonomy' has four closely related meanings"[3]: the "capacity" to govern one's self, the actual "condition" of self-government, an ideal character type, and as "the sovereign right of self-determination."[4] Dworkin's taxonomy of the uses of the term "autonomy" is more extensive:

> It [the term "autonomy"] is used sometimes as an equivalent of liberty (positive or negative in Berlin's terminology), sometimes as equivalent to self-rule or sovereignty, sometimes as identical with freedom of the will. It is equated with dignity, integrity, individuality, independence, responsibility, and self-knowledge. It is identified with qualities of self-assertion, with critical reflection, with absence of external causation, with knowledge of one's own interests.[5]

A similarly extensive taxonomy of uses of the term "autonomy" has been developed by Manuel Vargas, who, in reviewing Taylor's edited collection *Personal Autonomy*, noted that the term was used by the authors whose work was contained within that volume as:

> bare agency; a species of self-governed agency; a kind of relation to the world; an ideal of self-control that may rarely be had; a kind of rule-governed activity that is frequently had; ownership-taking for what one does; interchangeable with freedom; a conception of morally responsible agency; *neither* freedom nor morally responsible agency; competence for medical decision-making; authority over personal choices; self-rule; a designation for agents bound by political principles governing the basic

institutions of society; freedom from external influence; freedom from external control or restriction on choice; and, the kind of thing for which external restrictions on choice are largely irrelevant.[6]

Finally, an even more developed taxonomy of conceptions of autonomy has been offered by Nomy Arpaly, who identifies and discusses eight distinct accounts of autonomy in the literature: agent-autonomy, personal efficacy, independence of mind, normative moral autonomy, authenticity, self-identification, heroic autonomy, and reasons-responsiveness.[7]

Before moving to consider whether the concept of autonomy has as many faces as these taxonomies imply a note on the methodology of this chapter is in order. As was observed previously, the aim of this chapter is to show that autonomy is not as hydra-headed as it might first appear. To achieve this it will be noted that many of the ways in which "autonomy" is said to be understood cannot be held to be conceptions of personal autonomy at all (and so can be quickly rejected as such) for they clearly fail to capture the connotative contours of this concept. (Thus, for example, it will be noted almost in passing that Dworkin's view that on one conception of "autonomy" autonomy is coextensive with negative liberty is mistaken, for even nonautonomous agents could be negatively free.) Of course, many conceptions that are held to be conceptions of autonomy do not so clearly fail as such. In such cases one or more counterexamples to the conception at hand will be presented to support its rejection as a capturing analysis of autonomy. This approach might be understood as rather a dismissive one, but it is not intended to be. Rather, it is simply a version of the traditional analytical approach of showing that a conception of a concept is mistaken insofar as it fails to capture its connotative contours—albeit a version that is streamlined by having the connotative contours of the concept in question clearly outlined and to hand.[8] It should also be noted that the aim of this chapter is *not* to show that there is no philosophical value in the conceptions of autonomy that it will reject as analyses of personal autonomy. Rather, it is simply to note that they are not analyses of personal autonomy (and so there are not as many faces of this concept as it is usually believed), not that they are not philosophically interesting analyses in their own right of some *other* concept (such as, for example, identification). Thus, while they can be directly rejected as capturing analyses of personal autonomy, this does not imply that the arguments that have been developed to support them should not be directly engaged with by persons concerned with the concepts that they more closely capture.

## Feinberg's Taxonomy

Faced with the many different uses of the term "autonomy" it might be tempting to throw up one's hands in despair and retreat from the task of analyzing this concept. But this temptation should be resisted. It is clear that of the four conceptions of autonomy that Feinberg outlines only one can properly be called an account of autonomy as this term is used to capture the connotative contours outlined previously: "Autonomy as condition." The possession of the capacity for autonomy is simply the possession of having the capacity for the condition of autonomy, and so these are not distinct conceptions of autonomy at all. Similarly, Feinberg is clear that the conception of the autonomous person as one possessing an ideal complex of character traits will be drawn from the traits that he had earlier identified as being those involved in the condition of autonomy.[9] Rather than being a separate conception of autonomy, then, autonomy as an ideal is based upon autonomy as a condition. It is also clear that respecting autonomy as a right will be a normative response to the perceived value of autonomy as a condition. As John Christman notes, then, "nothing Feinberg says in his explication of the related manifestations of autonomy disturbs the claim that there is an important core upon which these related ideas rest (or grow out of)."[10]

## Dworkin's Taxonomy

It seems, however, that Christman's observation is inapplicable to Dworkin's taxonomy of conceptions of autonomy. This is because Dworkin's taxonomy, being both more extensive and more diverse, does not seem to possess any type of conceptual core, as did Feinberg's. The first point to note here is that Dworkin was right to observe that autonomy is sometimes taken to be identical with freedom of the will. However, as will be argued in Chapter 3, to assimilate these two concepts is a mistake, and so this so-called conception of autonomy can be put to one side until then. What, then, of the other qualities that Dworkin holds autonomy is understood to mean? Taking them in turn, it is not clear that Dworkin is correct to claim that autonomy is understood as negative liberty in Berlin's sense, where a person possesses negative liberty "to the degree to which no man or body of men interferes with . . . [her] . . . activity,"[11] for it is clear that even a wanton might possess this—and Dworkin cites no authors who explicitly equate autonomy and negative liberty in this way.[12] He is correct, however, to hold that autonomy is often taken to mean something similar to positive liberty, in Berlin's sense, where a person possesses positive liberty to the degree that she is "conscious of . . . [herself] . . . as a thinking, willing, active being, bearing responsibility for . . . [her] . . . choices and able to explain them by references to . . . [her] . . . own ideas and purposes."[13] As will be argued in Chapter 6, however, this assimilation of autonomy and positive liberty conflates claims about the ontology of autonomy with claims about its value to its possessors and so should be resisted. Dworkin is also correct to note that autonomy is often understood to be "equivalent to self-rule or sovereignty." This, though, should be taken as simply an etymological point rather than a philosophical one. Indeed, although almost every writer on autonomy would agree with this characterization of the concept, they would disagree with how one is to understand its constituent parts: what is the "self" that "rules," for example, and how is one to understand "sovereignty"? This understanding of autonomy, then, is really the starting point for an analysis of it, rather than a conception of it in itself.

What, then, of the other traits that Dworkin lists and that are understood as being conceptions of autonomy: dignity, integrity, individuality, independence, responsibility, self-knowledge, self-assertion, critical reflection, absence of external causation, and knowledge of one's own interests?[14] First, the non-Kantian account of personal autonomy that is of concern here does not carry with it the baggage associated with the concept of dignity, and so this term can be put to one side. Similarly, the association of the non-Kantian account of autonomy that is prominent in contemporary bioethics with responsibility can also be put to one side, for it is just not true that the concept of autonomy is uncritically used interchangeably with that of responsibility.[15] Second, it is not clear that all of these qualities are equated with personal autonomy, as Dworkin claims.[16] A child, for example, could both possess and exhibit individuality, independence, self-knowledge, self-assertion, be free from external causation, and know her own interests, but she could still fail to possess autonomy. And, as will be argued later in addressing Arpaly's account of autonomy as authenticity, an agent could possess integrity in that her actions are authentically hers, but she need not possess autonomy as this is generally understood. Finally, while it is true that many of these traits are often *associated* with personal autonomy, this does not show that they are *equated* with it, as Dworkin claims. Thus, that there might be many *aspects* of the connotative contours of this concept does not in itself show that there are an equal number of *conceptions* of it.

## Vargas's Taxonomy

Similar remarks can be made about Vargas's taxonomy of conceptions of autonomy, for it too can be significantly whittled down to a more manageable set of distinct accounts. First, Vargas is mistaken to hold that autonomy is understood as bare agency, except in rare cases—and then it is clear that the conception of autonomy that is in use is not that of *personal* autonomy, as this concept understood in both bioethics in particular and contemporary moral philosophy in general.[17] It is true that the possession of autonomy involves both "a species of self-governed agency," "self-rule," and "a kind of relation to the world," but, like Dworkin's noting that autonomy is associated with self-rule, these are not so much distinct characterizations of autonomy so much as they are core components of the concepts that could be accepted by all who use it. Also like Dworkin, Vargas is mistaken to claim that autonomy is held to be interchangeable with freedom.[18] He is correct, however, to note that the relationship between autonomy and morally responsible agency is a contested one—but this does not show that the participants in this debate therefore hold different conceptions of autonomy. Similarly, that there is a debate concerning the relationship between autonomy and the availability of choices and the imposition of restrictions does not show that the accounts of autonomy that its participants accept are necessarily distinct. Finally, Vargas is correct to note that autonomy has been variously characterized as " . . . an ideal of self-control that may rarely be had; a kind of rule-governed activity that is frequently had; ownership-taking for what one does; competence for medical decision-making; authority over personal choices . . . ". However, as will be discussed more extensively with respect to Arpaly's taxonomy of conceptions of autonomy, these observations do not show that autonomy is as hydra-headed a concept as it might first appear.[19]

## ARPALY'S TAXONOMY OF AUTONOMY

### Agent-autonomy

What, then, of Arpaly's taxonomy of differing conceptions of autonomy? As with Feinberg's, Dworkin's, and Vargas's, Arpaly's taxonomy of conceptions of autonomy transpires to be less extensive than it first appears. Arpaly begins her taxonomy of differing accounts of autonomy with one that she dubs "agent-autonomy." For Arpaly, "Agent-autonomy is a relationship between an agent and her motivational states that can be roughly characterized as the agent's ability to decide which of them to follow: it is a type of self-control or self-government that persons usually have and that nonhuman animals do not have."[20] Arpaly cites as proponents of accounts of agent-autonomy "the early Harry Frankfurt, Gary Watson, David Velleman, Robert Noggle, Michael Bratman, and Keith Lehrer," and notes that she has offered only "a very broad construal of agent-autonomy," for "different philosophers can agree that we . . . 'govern' ourselves while having very, very different views as to what constitutes this governing and as to which parts of a person, if any, constitute the 'governing' self and the 'governed' self."[21] One might, she notes, hold that "our autonomy is a matter of having second-order desires or that it is a matter of our having the ability to reflectively endorse actions, and so on . . . ."[22]

Although Arpaly is right to note that the accounts of so-called agent-autonomy that the previously named persons will provide will vary greatly, it is far from clear that she is correct in her supposition that these persons are all engaged with the same general project.[23] Be that as it may, even if we take at face value her claim that they are all pursuing the same project, it is also clear that even though these philosophers might use the term "autonomy," insofar as they are engaged on the Frankfurtian project of offering analyses of what it is for a person to identify with her motivational states they are not engaged in analyzing the concept of personal autonomy as this is generally understood.[24] As will be argued in Chapter 3, a person's identification with her effective first-order desires (i.e., her being "autonomous" with respect to them, where "autonomy" is here understood in the sense of agent-autonomy) is neither necessary nor sufficient for her to enjoy personal autonomy with respect to them. Accounts of so-called agent-autonomy, then, are thus not accounts of personal autonomy.

## Personal Efficacy

Having outlined so-called agent-autonomy Arpaly moves to outline a second, distinct, sense of autonomy: autonomy as personal efficacy.[25] Arpaly holds that persons who possess this type of autonomy will lack "various kinds of dependence on other people," for they are able "to get along well in the world without requiring the help of others."[26] On this sense of autonomy, writes Arpaly, "a person can make himself more autonomous by learning how to drive, becoming rich, becoming knowledgeable, or gaining physical strength."[27]

There are, unfortunately, many problems with this as an account of autonomy. First, it is not clear that this is an account of autonomy *per se*, so much as it is an account of what factors might make a person's autonomy more valuable for him. That is, just as Samson was not stronger when he breaks the new ropes that bound him but was simply more able to use his strength, so too it seems are persons not more autonomous when they are able to drive, or become wealthier, or stronger, but are simply more able to use their autonomy to fulfill their desires or pursue their goals. This criticism of the notion of autonomy as personal efficacy stems from the idea that the term "autonomy" refers to a capacity that persons have, rather than serving as a description of how they live their lives (e.g., autonomously, or not). That is, persons do not typically develop a greater capacity for autonomy when they learn to drive, or become wealthier, or stronger, but, instead, they are simply better able to utilize the capacity that they had.

Yet this initial criticism of the notion of autonomy as personal efficacy moves too quickly, for it implies that learning to drive, or becoming wealthier, or stronger, and so on, can aid a person only in exercising her preexisting capacity for autonomy. The relationship between the development of skills, and the acquiring of possessions or properties, and personal autonomy is, however, more complex than this. If, to be autonomous, a person must make her own decisions rather than abdicate her decision-making to others, she will need to trust her own judgment. If a person lacks such self-trust, she must, to be autonomous, develop it—and engaging in certain activities might aid her in doing so. For example, if a person who does not trust herself acquires a certain degree of wealth, she might begin to trust her own judgment as she exercises it as a consumer. Similarly, a person who is granted voting rights might begin to trust her judgment as she exercises them and discovers that she can defend her decisions and views against criticism. The development of skills and the acquisition of possessions or properties might thus enhance a person's capacity for autonomy through enabling her to develop traits that support its exercise. Such skills, possessions, or properties might thus enhance not only a person's *exercise* of autonomy but also her *capacity* for autonomy.[28] However, noting this does not lend any support to the notion of autonomy as personal efficacy. This is because, even though this is so, the increased independence that a person might possess as a result of (merely) having these skills, possessions, or properties is itself a form of autonomy. Rather, it is only the *expression* of her (possibly developing) autonomy. The possession of such skills, possessions, and properties thus still has only an instrumental relationship to autonomy and not a constitutive one—and it is this latter relationship that the proponents of the notion of autonomy as personal efficacy are committed to.

The understanding of autonomy as personal efficacy, then, is not one that could be accepted by anyone who accepts the connotative contours of personal autonomy as this concept is generally understood within contemporary bioethics and moral philosophy in general. Indeed, rather than being an account of autonomy per se, autonomy as personal efficacy seems to be more of an account of a way in which a person's autonomy could be valuable to him. Perhaps, though, the idea of personal efficacy as outlined by Arpaly could be partially constitutive of personal autonomy? But even this is doubtful. First, the enjoyment of personal efficacy is not necessary for a person to possess personal autonomy. To see this, consider the claims that on this view a person will be autonomous if she lacks "various kinds of dependence on other people," and has "the ability to get along well in the world without requiring the help of others." The proponents of this personal efficacy as autonomy would thus deem nonautonomous persons who pursue projects that necessarily require the aid of others, and who are accordingly dependent upon them. A person who wishes to beautify himself through cosmetic surgery, for example, will require the aid of a cosmetic surgeon, who in turn will require the aid of her surgical staff. But such dependence does not show that persons who undergo such surgery, or the surgeons who operate upon them, systematically suffer from a diminution in their autonomy. More generally, this account of autonomy would render anyone who was dependent upon others or required their aid less than fully autonomous—and this would include almost everyone but the most self-reliant of hermits. Shopkeepers, for example, depend upon their customers, customers depend upon their employers, and employers, in turn, depend upon *their* customers. Unless we are willing to accept that autonomy as personal efficacy comes close to being similar to the ideal of heroic autonomy that will be discussed next, it seems that autonomy as personal efficacy is not necessary for personal autonomy as this concept is generally understood.

Moreover, the enjoyment of personal efficacy is not sufficient for a person to be autonomous, either. Consider in this regard Anthony Fremont, the sinister child in Jerome Bixby's short story "It's a *Good* Life."[29] Anthony has the ability to control everything around him with his mind: the weather, what programs are shown on television, and the fate of every living thing around him. Anthony clearly does not depend on other people, nor does he need the help of others to get around in the world. Anthony, however, is the paradigm of the nonautonomous wanton. A willful small child, he does not reflect on his desires but simply acts upon them when they strike him. Personal efficacy is thus not only distinct from personal autonomy but its possession is neither necessary nor sufficient for a person to possess personal autonomy.

## Independence of Mind

What, then, of the third conception of autonomy that Arpaly identifies: autonomy as independence of mind? Unlike both agent-autonomy and autonomy as personal efficacy Arpaly does not, strictly speaking, characterize autonomy as independence of mind as being an understanding of autonomy, although she does include it in her taxonomy of "the various things that 'autonomy' means."[30] Instead, she simply notes that a person who lacks independence of mind, such as a person who (in Thomas E. Hill Jr.'s words) "blindly follows parental wishes, peer pressures, traditional norms, church authorities, or local fads, fashions, or folk heroes" would often be said to lack autonomy.[31] As such, then, unlike agent-autonomy or autonomy as personal efficacy, autonomy as independence of mind is not supposed to be an account of autonomy, but merely one trait that an autonomous person should possess.[32] Even so, the possession of this trait does not guarantee that its possessor is autonomous. Anthony Fremont, for example, clearly possesses independence of mind, and yet he is a nonautonomous wanton. More prosaically, a person who always thinks for herself might still suffer from a diminution in her autonomy with respect to her decisions, and consequently with respect to the actions that they lead her to perform, if another person has manipulated her into making them.

## Normative Moral Autonomy

Just as neither autonomy as personal efficacy nor autonomy as independence of mind are actually accounts of autonomy at all, nor is the third account of autonomy that Arpaly outlines.[33] According to Arpaly, "A further important notion of autonomy is the notion of *normative*, moral autonomy—the one invoked when people ask to be allowed to make their own decisions and to be free from paternalistic intervention."[34] Arpaly supports her claim that normative moral autonomy is an account of autonomy that is distinct from "the sense of 'autonomy' that autonomous-action theorists are looking for" with two examples.[35] In the first, "someone steals from you," but whereas the thief thereby "has violated your autonomy" it is plausible to claim that "you are no less an autonomous agent as a result: you are no less capable of governing your own actions than you were a moment ago."[36] In the second, a doctor lies to a patient or withholds information from him, "ignoring the fact that the patient is in the process of making an important employment decision to which his condition would be relevant."[37] In this case, Arpaly claims, "[m] any people" would hold that the doctor prevented his patient from making an autonomous decision. But, she goes on to claim, "This is ... obviously not the sense of 'autonomy' that autonomous-action theorists are looking for ... [for] ... Decisions made on incomplete or misleading data are everywhere ... [and so] to hold that such decisions are deficient in autonomy would seem to make autonomy too scarce a commodity ... "[38]

Arpaly uses these cases to support her view that normative moral autonomy is distinct from the account of autonomy that autonomous-action theorists are concerned with by holding that it shows that a person's normative moral autonomy could be violated without affecting this latter type of autonomy. At first sight, her use of the first of these cases is persuasive. It is certainly true that the thief has failed to respect his victim's autonomy by stealing from her, for in so doing he has made it plain that he will do as he wishes concerning her property irrespective of her views of the matter, whether she is autonomous with respect to them or not.[39] It is also true that in depriving her of her goods the thief has not thereby rendered his victim less autonomous with respect to her decisions or her actions than she would have otherwise been. This is because (as will be argued more fully in Chapter 7) whereas a person's economic situation might be relevant to the instrumental value of her autonomy to her it is not directly relevant to the question of how autonomous she is. The second example that Arpaly constructs in support of her position is, however, fatally flawed in two respects. Arpaly holds (rightly) that many people would think that the doctor in this example prevented his patient from making an autonomous decision. This is certainly correct, for lying to someone or withholding information from him are, as was noted in Chapter 1 when the connotative contours of the concept of autonomy were outlined, paradigmatic ways in which a person's autonomy with respect to her decisions and the actions that flow from them can be compromised by another person. However, she is wrong to hold that this is not the sense of "autonomy" that autonomy theorists are looking for on the grounds that if it were autonomy would be overly scarce since decisions made on incomplete or misleading data are legion. This is because Arpaly is wrong to hold that autonomy theorists are committed to claiming that persons who make their decisions on "incomplete or misleading data" thereby suffer from a lack of autonomy. Persons who believe that the doctor in Arpaly's second example precluded his patient from making an autonomous decision would believe that this was so because he *deceived* him (either by commission or omission), and thereby led him to make a decision that he would not have otherwise made. In this situation, then, it was the doctor, and not the patient, who was directing the decisions that he was making. As such, then, the patient's autonomy with respect to his decisions was compromised *not* by the mere fact that the data he based them on were "incomplete or misleading," but by the fact that it was *deliberately* withheld from him or used to mislead him. Thus, one could *both* hold that this doctor compromised his patient's autonomy *and* hold that the type of autonomy that was thus compromised was the agent-autonomy that is of interest to autonomy theorists, *without* thereby committing oneself to the view that the possession of autonomy is an uncommon occurrence.

Yet even if Arpaly is mistaken to believe that her second example shows that normative moral autonomy is distinct from "the sense of 'autonomy' that autonomous-action theorists are looking for" (and hence is a distinctive form of autonomy in its own right) it was noted previously that her first example is persuasive at first sight—and so does not this show that she is correct to hold that normative moral autonomy is a distinct type of autonomy? (Recall here that Arpaly only needs one example in which normative moral autonomy is clearly distinct from autonomous-action theorists' view of autonomy to prove her case.) It does not. To see this, note that this example shows only that A can legitimately complain that B has failed to respond to A's autonomy in a morally appropriate way *even if* the acts of B that A is complaining about did not compromise the form of A's autonomy that Arpaly takes to be of interest to autonomy theorists. From the legitimacy of such a complaint Arpaly (implicitly) infers that some form of autonomy *other than* this form of A's autonomy must have been compromised. If she does not make this inference then this example will not support her claim that normative moral autonomy is distinct from this type of autonomy. This is because, absent this inference, all that this example shows is that B can fail to respect this type of autonomy of A without thereby compromising it—a point that, as discussed next, is perfectly comprehensible without invoking a distinct form of autonomy that is separable from the form of A's autonomy that Arpaly takes to be of interest to autonomy theorists. Yet Arpaly's inference is only justified if one assumes that A's complaint that B has failed to respond to his autonomy in the morally appropriate manner is *only* legitimate if this failure has resulted in (some form of) A's autonomy being compromised. But not only does Arpaly provide no argument in favor of this implicit premise, it is clearly not one that should be accepted. This is because it is perfectly possible for B to fail to respect the autonomy of A in a manner that could support A having a legitimate moral complaint against B on the grounds that she failed to respect her autonomy, even though B's actions did *not* compromise A's autonomy. As noted already, Arpaly's own example of the thief (B) and his victim (A) shows this clearly. (Although here A will have other grounds for complaint about B!) However, if one is not (yet) convinced that a person's economic situation is irrelevant to her autonomy with respect to her decisions or actions, consider the character of Frederick Clegg in John Fowles' novel *The Collector*. After winning a large sum of money in the football pools Clegg, a butterfly collector, buys an isolated farmhouse and kidnaps

Miranda Grey, an art student who he has admired from a distance, hoping that she will eventually fall in love with him. Eventually, Miranda becomes seriously ill and dies. Clegg considers suicide, but after reading Miranda's diary and realizing her true (and negative) feelings for him decides that he is better off without her. As the novel ends, Clegg is plotting to kidnap another girl. It is clear that Clegg has no respect for the autonomy of his victims—but it is equally clear that their autonomy was not compromised until he actually kidnapped them.[40] Arpaly's implicit premise—that A's complaint that B has failed to respond to his autonomy in the morally appropriate manner is *only* legitimate if this failure has resulted in (this form of) A's autonomy being compromised—should thus be rejected, for A could legitimately issue this complaint against B even though his autonomy is inviolate. Since this is so, neither of Arpaly's two examples succeed in showing that there is a form of autonomy called "normative moral autonomy" that is distinct from autonomous-action autonomy. The first fails because the implicit premise that was needed for her example to show this should be rejected, and the second fails because it is based on a misunderstanding of what forms of "incomplete or misleading" information can serve to compromise the autonomy of those who act on them. As such, then, Arpaly has only shown that a person's autonomy could fail to be respected even if it is not compromised—a position that is perfectly compatible with there being only *one* account of autonomy.

Yet although these arguments against Arpaly's view that normative moral autonomy is distinct from the form of autonomy that autonomous-action theorists are interested in might seem conclusive Arpaly has a ready response to them: that the type of autonomy that is of primary interest to autonomous-action theorists and that is thus, on her view, distinct from normative moral autonomy is not properly characterized in the previous responses to her arguments. Arpaly could note that the type of autonomy that she is here contrasting normative moral autonomy with is *agent-autonomy*—and that agent-autonomy is clearly distinct from the type of autonomy that is held to be of interest to autonomous-action theorists in the previous responses.[41] To see this, recall that persons who are concerned with normative moral autonomy would hold that a deceived patient would suffer from compromised autonomy as a result of being deceived. As will be argued in Chapter 3, however, a person concerned with agent-autonomy (i.e., identification) would *not* hold that a person's identifications with his desires would be compromised by deception. As such, it seems that Arpaly is right to hold that normative moral autonomy and agent-autonomy are distinct concepts—and thus right to hold that normative moral autonomy is a distinct understanding of autonomy in its own right.[42]

Yet this argument moves too quickly. To be sure, it shows that normative moral autonomy and agent-autonomy are distinct. But this should come as no surprise, for, as was noted previously, agent-autonomy is not coextensive with personal autonomy. Thus, showing that normative moral autonomy (i.e., that account of personal autonomy on which a person's autonomy could be compromised through his being successfully deceived) and agent-autonomy (i.e., identification) are distinct does *not*, as Arpaly believes, show that the former is a distinct conception of personal autonomy in its own right, and one that is different from that of agent-autonomy understood as another account of autonomy.[43] Rather, it just reinforces the point (made briefly above, and more fully in Chapter 3) that so-called agent-autonomy is not really an account of autonomy at all.

In brief, then, if the sense of autonomy that Arpaly takes autonomous-action theorists to be concerned with is understood as that which captures the connotative contours of this concept as these are outlined in Chapter 1, then Arpaly's two examples fail to show that this is distinct from normative moral autonomy. Her first example only shows that a person can fail to respect a person's autonomy without thereby compromising it, which is compatible with there being only one account of autonomy at issue, and her second is fatally flawed, for it is based on a misunderstanding of the relationship between a person's autonomy with respect to her decisions and the data on which she made them. If, however, the sense of autonomy that Arpaly takes autonomous-action theorists to be concerned with is understood as agent-autonomy (which seems to be the case), then it is not surprising that normative moral autonomy is distinct from agent-autonomy, for agent-autonomy is not an account of personal autonomy at all. In either case, then, Arpaly has failed to support her claim that the sense of autonomy that autonomous-action theorists are concerned with is a form of autonomy that is distinct from normative moral autonomy.

## Autonomy as Authenticity

While there is thus considerable reason to doubt that the first four senses of autonomy that Arpaly outlines in her taxonomy of the contemporary uses of this term are even accounts of autonomy, let alone accounts of personal autonomy as this is generally understood within the literature, the fifth sense of autonomy that she outlines undoubtedly satisfies the first of these two desiderata. This is because the sense of autonomy as authenticity has been developed by Harry Frankfurt—and, unlike his analysis of identification, Frankfurt's account of autonomy as authenticity is undoubtedly intended to be an analysis of autonomy.[44]

According to Frankfurt, "A person acts autonomously only when his volitions derive from the essential character of his will."[45] As Velleman notes, this account of autonomy has, at first sight, strong Kantian overtones.[46] Frankfurt, however, takes pains to distinguish his account of autonomy from that of Kant. Noting that the autonomous will is, for Kant, one that "is entirely devoid of all empirical motives, preferences, and desires," and so "is identical in everyone," Frankfurt stresses that persons will, on his account of autonomy, be autonomous when they are motivated to act by "their contingent personal features" that make them "distinctive and that characterize their specific identities."[47] Given this, for Frankfurt, a person will be fully autonomous when she is moved by either the volitional necessity of performing a certain action, or when she refrains from acting when she realizes that the action is unthinkable for her. To illustrate volitional necessity Frankfurt draws upon Martin Luther's famous declaration "Here I stand; I can do no other."[48] Here, Frankfurt writes, Luther is constrained to act in a certain way by his own will, which motivates him to act in a way that not only is he unwilling to oppose, but that "his unwillingness is itself something which he is unwilling to alter."[49] Similarly, when a person is motivated to refrain from an action because it is unthinkable to him, "His inability to go through with the action reveals it as one that he is unwilling to will."[50] To illustrate this latter point Frankfurt offers the example of Lord Fawn, who, in Trollope's *The Eustace Diamonds*, cannot bring himself to converse with his estate-steward, Andy Gowran, about his, Fawn's, fiancée's infidelity, an act of which Gowran witnessed, after Gowran winked at him while recounting the event. At this point, even though he had resolved to find out about his fiancée's actions from Gowran, Fawn discovered that he was "unwilling for his will to be shaped" in the way that this would require; "He found that he simply could not do it."[51] On Frankfurt's understanding of autonomy, then, both Luther and Fawn were fully autonomous when they were moved to act, or to refrain from acting, by being compelled to do so through volitional necessity and unthinkability.

Frankfurt's understanding of autonomy here has been trenchantly criticized by Velleman, who holds that being governed in these ways by one's "motivational essence" "might amount to authenticity, perhaps, but not autonomy."[52] To show this, Velleman considers "the paradigm case of inauthenticity, the person who manifests what D. W. Winnicott called a 'False Self'."[53] The person who has a "False Self" "laughs at what he thinks he is supposed to find amusing, shows concern for what he thinks he is supposed to care about, and in general conforms himself to the demands and expectations of others."[54] The motive that this person has for behaving in this way is to satisfy others' expectations, and yet he neither acknowledges this as his motive, nor does he endorse it. It is thus not part of his essential nature, as this is construed by Frankfurt. Yet, although this person is not acting authentically, he is not lacking in autonomy. Indeed, argues Velleman, this person's "grip on the reins of his behavior is too tight, not too loose," with his inauthenticity stemming from not too little autonomy, but too much.[55]

Velleman's criticism of Frankfurt's understanding of autonomy as authenticity is plausible. However, it is not clear that the person who manifests a "False Self" is as much a paradigm of inauthenticity as Velleman believes. Velleman's case against Frankfurt's view rests on the intuition that a person who governs himself as the person with a "False Self" does acts inauthentically. It is not hard to see why we would believe this. After all, this person's acts are, in an obvious sense, inauthentic; his laughter does not indicate genuine amusement, his romantic gestures do not indicate genuine love, and his outbursts do not indicate genuine anger. However, it is not obvious that we can assume from the fact that his acts were inauthentic in the sense of not representing what this person genuinely felt that he was not acting authentically, in the sense of acting from who he really was, when he performed them. If this person was someone who always took all of his behavioral cues from others it is not implausible to hold his actions were representative of who he really was; they represented his nature as an other-directed cipher. As such, while his laughter might not be authentic in the sense of its expressing genuine amusement, it would be authentic in the sense of being representative of this person's other-directedness. It would be authentically inauthentic. If this is possible, then insofar as this person could not help but act in this way owing to his other-directed nature, and insofar as this coincides with his exhibiting a high degree of self-control, we should be led to praise Frankfurt's account of autonomy, not to bury it.

Yet although Velleman's criticism of Frankfurt's understanding of autonomy can be met in this way, this might still only give cold comfort to those who accept Frankfurt's view here. The example of the authentically inauthentic person that was offered as an initial defense of Frankfurt's position proves to be its undoing. For this example to work against Velleman all that needs to be true is that the agent in question is authentically inauthentic; that is, he is authentically other-directed. It does not, however, need to be the case that this agent is actually a *person*, in Frankfurt's sense of the term. He could, instead, simply be a mere (and nonautonomous) agent—someone who responds in this way to the expectations of others without either considering why he does this, or caring that he does so. Such an agent would exhibit all of the outward characteristics of Winnicott's "False Self," but he would not do so because he was exhibiting a high degree of self-control, as Velleman holds. Instead, he would simply be reacting to what he perceived his situation to be, as a fox might respond to the sight of a rabbit. Instead of accepting Velleman's criticism of Frankfurt's understanding of autonomy, then, we could instead posit one that is its mirror image: an agent might be fully authentic, in that his actions flow from his motivational essence, but still fail to be autonomous—and so autonomy and authenticity are not coextensive, as Frankfurt believes.

This objection to Frankfurt's view might, however, have moved too quickly. It appears that the understanding of authenticity that Frankfurt is concerned with is related to a person's being subject to either volitional necessity or unthinkability. As such, it seems that a mere agent cannot act authentically in Frankfurt's sense of the term, for he will lack the reflexive attitude towards his will, which is the hallmark of being constrained in the requisite ways. But to offer this response on behalf of Frankfurt's views would to be to overlook the fact that when Lord Fawn broke off his conversation with Gowran—an act that Frankfurt held to be an authentic one—his having to do so came as a surprise to him. As such, Lord Fawn had clearly not adopted any reflexive attitudes towards his will prior to being so moved by it—and so his motivational structure at the point at which he initially acted would be no different with respect to this particular action that would be that of a mere (nonautonomous) agent. Given this, then, it seems that the prior objection to Frankfurt's understanding of autonomy as authenticity stands. Authenticity and autonomy are distinct concepts.[56]

## Autonomy as Self-identification

A person who is moved by volitional necessity or unthinkability, or both, would not experience the motivational forces that constrain her as being alien to her. From this, Arpaly outlines a further understanding of autonomy—autonomy as self-identification.[57] A person who possesses this type of autonomy will be a person "with a harmonious and coherent self-image who never experiences her desires as an external threat."[58] Such a person would not, for example, be in the situation of "a woman who has the sudden urge to drown her bawling child in the bath . . . or . . . [of] . . . a squash player who, while suffering an ignominious defeat, desires to smash his opponent in the face with the racket," and who desires these things "in spite of themselves."[59] That is, such a person would never be beset by external desires but would only act upon desires that she believed were truly her own.

On Arpaly's (brief) account of what it is for a person to possess this sort of autonomy it is not clear how much, if at all, it is supposed to differ from so-called agent-autonomy. Indeed, Arpaly introduces her discussion of autonomy as self-identification by outlining Frankfurt's early metaphors for what it is for a person to identify with a desire, on which an effective first-order desire that she feels "passive" with respect to, and which she experiences as "external" to her, is one that she is alienated from, rather than identifies with.[60] And if autonomy as self-identification simply is so-called agent-autonomy, then the criticism that so-called agent-autonomy (i.e., identification) should not be conflated with personal autonomy proper that was outlined previously (and that will be fully developed in Chapter 3) will apply here too. Yet even if there is a substantive (if elusive) difference between autonomy as self-identification and so-called agent-autonomy, it is clear that insofar as it focuses upon a person's subjective view of his own motivations autonomy as self-identification will fail to capture the connotative contours of the concept of personal autonomy as these are widely understood. Such a subjective conception of autonomy will be unable to account for a person's suffering from a diminution in his autonomy with respect to his decisions, and hence with respect to the actions that they motivate him to perform, when he is unknowingly subjected to successful interpersonal manipulation. Othello, for example, might well have failed to experience his desire to smother Desdemona as one that was alien to him, but he nonetheless suffered from diminished autonomy with respect to it to the extent that his performance of it was under the control of Iago. Like the conceptions of autonomy that preceded it in Arpaly's taxonomy, then, autonomy as self-identification is not an account of personal autonomy as this is generally understood.

## Heroic Autonomy

The seventh conception of autonomy that Arpaly identifies is heroic autonomy. Such an account of autonomy might encompass "ideals such as Spinoza's freedom, stoic apathia or ataraxia, Aristotle's life of contemplation, Freud's or Jung's ideals of the liberation that their methods were to aim at bringing, Nietzsche's idea of the free spirit, and other states that are supposed to be desirable and only attainable by the few."[61] It is, however, generally understood that most adult humans have the capacity for personal autonomy, and so this heroic ideal is, at best, a conception of autonomy that is distinct from that which is of concern in bioethics and moral philosophy.[62]

## Autonomy as Responsiveness to Reasons

The last view of autonomy that Arpaly considers is that a person is autonomous if she acts for reasons that she endorses. As Arpaly observes, this is because "Rational and reason-responsive action is thought of as requiring deliberation or endorsement, and autonomous actions are also often regarded as the result of deliberation or endorsement. . . Things that impair our ability to respond to reasons, such as alcohol and hypnosis, are supposed to impair our autonomy. Animals are often said not to respond to reasons, and they are often said not to be autonomous."[63] By themselves, these are not good reasons to assimilate reasons-responsiveness to personal autonomy. That P requires X, and Q requires X too, does not show that P and Q are coextensive. Similarly, that Y impairs both P and Q does not show that P and Q are coextensive. With the above quoted observation in hand, however, Arpaly observes that there is generally understood to be a close connection between reasons-responsiveness and autonomy.[64] Having noted this supposed connection, however, Arpaly argues that those who accept it are mistaken. Arpaly holds that "acting for reasons, including acting rationally, is not necessarily related to agent-endorsement or to deliberation," and so it is not obvious "that intuitions about self-control and agent-endorsement belong with intuitions about rationality and responsiveness to reasons."[65] In brief, Arpaly believes that acting for reasons is not necessarily related to deliberation because a person could act for reasons without deliberating. To support this claim she offers examples of what she terms "fast action"—actions that the person performing them does not deliberate about, but simply does—such as those performed by an accomplished tennis player during a fast-paced game. Arpaly holds that we can legitimately judge such a tennis player's fast actions as either rational (we praise them), or irrational (we criticize them).[66] If Arpaly is right here, and if it is the case that autonomy is connected with deliberation, and reasons-responsiveness is not, then she will be correct to hold that autonomy is not connected with reasons-responsiveness, either.

There are, however, two responses that can be made to this argument for Arpaly's assertion that persons can be praised or blamed for their fast actions can be criticized on two fronts. First, the attribution of praise or blame to persons on the basis of their fast actions is not as clear-cut as Arpaly believes. We might praise the fast actions of an accomplished tennis player, to be sure, but it is not obvious that such praise is anything more than aesthetic appreciation of her actions, as we might similarly praise the fast actions of an accomplished gymnast—and such approval does not imply that we believe that the actions performed are either rational or irrational. Second, and on a related note, it seems that persons are *not* praised or blamed for the rationality or otherwise of their fast actions. Instead, typically persons disavow that such actions are subject to tests of rationality by saying that they were performed "in the heat of the moment," and hence not subject to the usual attributions of rationality or irrationality. (A position that is consistent, of course, with accepting that persons might take the fast actions of others to be indicative of the moral character of the person who performed them, just as they might accept the similar evidentiary power of Freudian slips.) As such, then, Arpaly has not shown that reasons-responsiveness is unconnected to autonomy.

## CONCLUSION

It was argued in this chapter that there are fewer varieties of autonomy in the philosophical literature than might at first appear. Feinberg failed to show that there are four distinct conceptions of autonomy, while both Dworkin and Vargas failed to establish their extensive taxonomies of conceptions of autonomy. And of the eight accounts of autonomy that Arpaly identifies only two (reasons-responsiveness and autonomy as authenticity) are conceptions of autonomy that are related to personal autonomy as this is generally understood. The others either transpire not be accounts of autonomy at all, but of some other concept entirely (i.e., agent-autonomy, and its twin, autonomy as self-identification), or they are accounts not of autonomy itself, but of a trait that is included within the concept of autonomy (i.e., independence of mind), or of ways that it is appropriate to respond to autonomy (i.e., normative moral autonomy), or they are simply unconnected with the contemporary understanding of autonomy as *personal* autonomy (i.e., personal efficacy, heroic autonomy).

The concept of autonomy, then, does not have as many faces as it might seem to have at first. Thus, even though the analysis of practical autonomy that was developed in the previous chapter was a partially stipulative one, since it is a capturing account of autonomy it can legitimately lay claim to be a (if not *the*) core account of autonomy for use in contemporary moral philosophy—and especially those contemporary discussions of bioethics in which this concept plays a central role. To lend further support to this claim it will be argued in the next chapter that autonomy and identification ("agent-autonomy," in Arpaly's terminology) are distinct concepts.

# 3 Identification and Autonomy
## A Tale of Two Concepts

## INTRODUCTION

Since the publication of Harry Frankfurt's seminal essay "Freedom of the Will and the Concept of a Person" it has been the best of times and the worst of times for philosophers who work on, or with, the concept of autonomy.[1] It is clear why the years since the publication of that essay have been the best of times for autonomy theory. As noted in the Introduction, "Freedom of the Will and the Concept of a Person" stimulated a significant interest in the question of what conditions must be met for an agent to possess the sort of freedom that is peculiar to persons, that which a person has when "he is free to want what he wants to want."[2] Many philosophers have taken this to be the question of what conditions must be met for a person to be autonomous, and so "Freedom of the Will and the Concept of a Person" stimulated a great deal of discussion of the nature of autonomy. Moreover, as was also noted in the Introduction, this burgeoning interest in the concept of autonomy has both stimulated, and been stimulated by, the increasingly central role that autonomy has come to play in many areas of bioethics, ranging from clinically orientated discussions concerning the nature of informed consent to the more policy-orientated debates concerning organ procurement and the use of reproductive technologies.[3] Yet although the influence of Frankfurt's essay can be used to explain (at least in part) why this is the best of times for persons who work on, or with, the concept of autonomy, it can also be used to explain why it is also now the worst of times for them. In "Freedom of the Will and the Concept of a Person" Frankfurt aimed to develop an account of what it is for a person to "identify with" her effective first-order desires—those desires that moved her to act or to refrain from acting. For Frankfurt, the question of what it is for a person to identify with her first-order desires was the key to answering the question of what is required for a person to act freely and of her own free will—a question that is related to the question of what it is for a person to enjoy freedom of the will.[4] The questions that Frankfurt was addressing, then, are *metaphysical* questions. That is, they are questions whose answers depend solely upon the nature of free will and the structure of the universe in which the person whose free will is in question finds herself. However, as was clear in the development of the account of practical autonomy in Chapter 1, the question of whether a person is autonomous with respect to her decisions and her actions is a *political* question. That is, it is a question whose answer depends on how a person's decisions and actions have been affected by her interactions with other agents. The metaphysical concept of identification is thus not synonymous with the political concept of autonomy.[5] The success of Frankfurt's 1971 essay in stimulating interest in autonomy theory has thus led to a systematic confusion between the concepts of autonomy and identification—a confusion that has been detrimental to the analysis of both.[6]

The primary aim of this chapter, then, is to show that the concepts of identification and autonomy are not coextensive. As will become clear below, differentiating the concepts of identification and autonomy is crucial for those discussions in bioethics that draw upon the latter concept, for, unless it is differentiated from that of identification, they will be faced with several serious theoretical difficulties—not the least of which being the charge that the concept of autonomy is simply irrelevant to debates in bioethics. To achieve the primary aim of this chapter, a brief analysis of the denotations of the concept of identification will be provided. Although this will not be a complete analysis of this concept (this will be provided in the next chapter), it will (given the analysis of practical autonomy that was developed in Chapter 1) suffice to show that the concepts of identification and autonomy are distinct. With this distinction in place, the secondary aim of this chapter is to show that the failure to distinguish these two concepts has had deleterious effects both on the analyses of them that have been developed and on the discussions within bioethics in which autonomy plays a central role. Finally, this chapter will conclude by addressing the contrary claim that identification and autonomy are not distinct concepts but are simply two conceptions of the same concept—and that this overarching concept can be termed either "autonomy" or "identification."

## SOURCES OF CONFUSION

Prior to turning to distinguish between the concepts of identification and autonomy it would be useful to outline the reasons why they are taken to be coextensive with each other. The first reason is simply a historical one. Frankfurt's original account of identification was developed at around the same time as Gerald Dworkin's influential account of autonomy, and the questions that Frankfurt and Dworkin were addressing have strong surface similarities. Frankfurt was addressing the question of what conditions must be met for a person to act freely and of his own free will, while Dworkin was addressing the question of what conditions must be met for a person to

enjoy self-rule.[7] Moreover, both Frankfurt and Dworkin offered hierarchi-
cally based answers to their respective questions. For Frankfurt, a person
acts freely and of his own free will when he has a second-order desire that
his first-order desire be effective in moving him to act. In forming such a second-order volition, Frankfurt writes, the person will have *identified himself*
with his effective first-order desire[8]; he will have "made this will his own."[9]

Similarly, on Dworkin's early theory of autonomy, "which may be characterized, in desperate brevity, by the formula autonomy = authenticity +
independence," for a person to be autonomous with respect to those of his
"decisions, motives, desires, habits, and so forth" that move him to act they
must be authentic; the person who is moved by them must view them as
"his."[10] For Dworkin, "It is the attitude a person takes towards the influences
motivating him which determines whether or not they are to be considered
'his.' Does he identify with them, assimilate them to himself, view himself as
the kind of person who wishes to be motivated in these particular ways?"[11]

Both Frankfurt and Dworkin, then, make the question of whether a person endorses his effective motivations crucial to answering their respective
questions of whether he acts freely and of his own free will, or of whether he
is autonomous with respect to his actions. Moreover, in addition to the similarities of the questions that Frankfurt and Dworkin address, and the simi-
larity of the answers that they give to them, they both explicitly state that the
central issue that they are concerned with is that of whether a person *identifies himself* with his effective motivations. Given these three important similarities between Frankfurt's early work on identification and Dworkin's early
work on autonomy it is not surprising that they have been widely taken to be
addressing the same issue. It is thus not surprising that the question of what
conditions must be met for a person to identify with his effective first-order
desires is also widely taken to be the question of what conditions must be met
for him to be autonomous with respect to them. Indeed, so widespread is the
view that Frankfurt and Dworkin have offered substantially similar analyses
of the same concept that it is common for persons to write of the "Frankfurt–
Dworkin" approach to analyzing identification, or autonomy, with the terms
"autonomy" and "identification" being used interchangeably.[12]

This historical reason for why the concepts of identification and autonomy
are treated as coextensive provides, however, only a partial explanation of
their widespread assimilation. Another reason why these concepts are treated
in this way is that the type of decision procedure that a person is held to
undergo prior to identifying with an effective first-order desire is, intuitively,
the same as that which she is held to undergo prior to being autonomous with
respect to it. It is, for example, intuitive to hold that a person will identify
with a first-order desire, that it is truly his own, if, given the situation that
he is in, it is a desire that he both wants to have and wants to be moved by,
just as it is intuitive to think that these criteria must be met for him to be
autonomous with respect to it.[13] As such, it is intuitive to think that a person's
identification with her effective first-order desire simply is what is involved

in her being autonomous with respect to it. Similarly, just as the concepts of identification and autonomy appear to be indistinguishable with respect to the decision-making procedures that persons must engage in for them to be applicable to their desires, so, too, do they seem to share certain defeating conditions. If a person is coerced into performing a certain action, for example, it would intuitively seem to be mistaken to claim that he had performed it freely and of his own free will. A person's being coerced into acting, then, seems to preclude her identification with the effective first-order desire that moved her to act.[14] Similarly, it would intuitively seem to be mistaken to claim that a person was autonomous with respect to an action that he was coerced into doing. Coercion, then, seems to be a defeating condition for both identification and autonomy. Unendorsed addiction also appears to be a defeating condition for both a person's identification with his effective first-order (addictive) desires, as well as for his autonomy with respect to them. Intuitively, if an addict acts on an addictive desire that he did not want to act on, he acted neither freely and of his free will. Nor, it seems, would such an addict be autonomous with respect to the actions that he performed in satisfying his unwanted addictive desire, since in acting to satisfy it he would not be directing himself to act in the way that he wishes.[15] Finally, it appears that a person's weakness of will would defeat both her ability to act freely and of her own free will, and her autonomy with respect to her effective first-order desires. A person who acts on a desire that she believes she has less reason to act on than another, competing, desire would not be moved to act by that desire that she endorses, that she identifies with. Similarly, a person who is moved to act through weakness of will is not ruling herself, so much as being subject to the rule of her (literally) unruly desires—and so to the extent that this is so she will suffer from a lack of autonomy with respect to her effective (but weak-willed) desires. Coercion, addiction, and weakness of the will all appear to be defeating conditions for both a person's identification with her effective first-order desires and her autonomy with respect to them insofar as they work to prevent a person from directing her actions as she wishes. These conditions thus appear to be defeating conditions for *both* concepts for the *same* reasons. As such, it is not surprising that in discussions of the effects that these phenomena have upon a person's identification with her effective first-order desires, or her autonomy with respect to them, a person's ability to act freely and of her own free will and her ability to act autonomously have been treated as though they were coextensive.

## IDENTIFICATION AND AUTONOMY: DISTINCT CONCEPTS

### Identification is Not Sufficient for Autonomy

Coercion, addiction, and weakness of will are all generally agreed to be defeating conditions for both identification and autonomy, and, as such, appear to support the view that these are coextensive concepts. However, one defeating condition for autonomy is conspicuous by its absence on this list: interpersonal manipulation. It is clear that the successful manipulation of a person into performing an action that she would not have otherwise performed would serve to compromise the manipulee's autonomy with respect to her manipulated actions. As noted in Chapter 1, when Iago manipulated Othello into performing the actions that culminated in the death of Desdemona, it was Iago, and not Othello, who was actually directing Othello's actions. Othello was a mere marionette in the hands of Iago, who was tweaking and twitching upon his motivational strings to direct him to perform the actions that he, Iago, wanted him to perform. Since it was thus Iago, and not Othello, who was directing Othello's actions, Othello lacked self-direction, and thus autonomy, with respect to them. But that Othello lacked autonomy with respect to the actions that he performed only as a result of Iago's manipulations does not show that he therefore also failed to identify with them. Indeed, on Frankfurt's account of identification Othello certainly performed the actions that Iago manipulated him into performing freely and of his own free will. Othello did "what he wanted to do . . . he did it because he wanted to do it, and . . . the will by which he was moved when he did it was his will because it was the will he wanted."[16] Moreover, "Even supposing that he could have done otherwise, he would not have done otherwise; and even supposing that he could have had a different will, he would not have wanted his will to differ from what it was."[17] And "since the will that moved him when he acted was his will because he wanted it to be, he cannot claim that his will was forced upon him or that he was a passive bystander to its constitution."[18]

That Othello acts freely and of his own free will when he is manipulated by Iago and yet suffers from a diminution in his autonomy with respect to both his effective first-order desires and the actions that they move him to perform shows that a person's identification with his effective first-order desires is not sufficient for him to be autonomous with respect to either them, or the actions that they move him to perform.[19] And this should not be surprising, especially once one considers how interpersonal manipulation operates. Iago manipulated Othello through having both intimate knowledge of his desires and values and the ability to control the information that he had access to such that he could control what he believed. Thus armed, he was able to manipulate the information that Othello received so that he could bring him to hold certain beliefs that, when combined with his desires, would lead him to form certain effective first-order desires, and thence to act in certain ways. Iago, then, led Othello to form those effective first-order desires that he wanted him to form through manipulating his ability to make decisions and form effective first-order desires on the basis of his beliefs and preexisting desires and values. The structure and operation of Othello's will when he forms these effective first-order desires is, *ex hypothesi, identical* to that which he would have were he not to be manipulated by Iago (i.e., were Iago only to be presenting him with the facts as he saw them, with no ulterior motive for so doing). Thus, since the question of whether Othello acts freely and of his own free will rests on the way in which his will is structured, that he is subject to interpersonal manipulation of this sort is *irrelevant* to the question of whether he acts freely and of his own free will. However, as was argued in Chapter 1 the question of whether a person has been manipulated into making certain decisions, and hence performing certain actions, is *not* irrelevant to the question of whether she was autonomous with respect to those decisions or those actions. This is because such information is crucial to answer the question of whether it was he, or someone else, who was directing her decisions and her actions. Thus, a person who is successfully subject to interpersonal manipulation might still act freely and of his own free will, but he will not act autonomously.

## A Brief Sketch of an Analysis of Identification

Just as identifying with one's effective first-order desires is not sufficient for one to be autonomous with respect to them, it is not necessary, either. To show this, a brief account of what it is for a person to identify with her effective first-order desires is needed. This account will be developed further in the next chapter, and will supplement, rather than supplant, Frankfurt's original hierarchical account of identification that was outlined previously.[20]

Any account of identification must meet three conditions. First, it must be able to distinguish between the effective first-order desires that are held by persons and by nonpersons. Second, it must be able to distinguish between those effective first-order desires that a person possesses *qua* person, and those that she merely possesses *qua* agent. Finally, any account of identification must be, in Dworkin's phrase, judgmentally relevant.[21] That is, it must satisfy standard pre-theoretical intuitions concerning when a person does, and when she does not, act freely and of her own free will—or, if it does not, be able to provide the basis for a plausible justification as to why such intuitions should be jettisoned.

With these criteria in hand a brief account of what it is for a person to identify with her effective first-order desires can be outlined. The first point to note is a simple one. Analyses of identification are analyses of what it is for *persons* (i.e., agents for whom the question of whether their wills are free is a relevant one) to identify with their effective first-order desires. Analyses of identification thus must require that certain criteria be met for a person to identify with her effective first-order desires that could *only* be met by persons. And, as Frankfurt rightly points out, it is an essential characteristic of persons that they can want certain first-order desires to be effective in moving them to action. To capture this feature of persons the analysis of identification that will be developed in this volume (and, in brief, here) will be a hierarchical account, on which it will be necessary for a person to identify with one of his effective first-order desires that he endorse it in some way. Moreover, since a person cannot passively endorse a desire, but, instead, must *decide* to do so, the account of identification that will be developed in this volume will be an account of *decisive* identification.[22]

On this account of identification, then, any effective first-order desire that a person identifies with will be related to his individual motivational-set in such a way that he could endorse it. Yet although this requirement might appear trivially to follow from those outlined previously, articulating it serves the useful purpose of bringing to light the fact that there are two ways in which a person's first-order desires might be endorsable by a person, given his preexisting motivational-set. They might be endorsable insofar as they are in accord with desires within his motivational-set that he shares with (almost) every other agent, whether the agent is a person or not. Such "agential" desires would be, for example, the desire to avoid pain, the desire to remain alive, or the desires to alleviate hunger or thirst. Alternatively, an agent's first-order desires might be endorsable by elements of his existing motivational-set insofar as they are desires that accord with its own peculiar configuration, and which need not accord with the configurations of motivational-sets possessed by other agents. The "personal" desires to go train spotting, or cross-country skiing, would not, for example, be endorsable by the motivational-sets of (almost) all agents. Insofar as analyses of identification are analyses of what it is for a *person* to identify with her desires (since only persons can enjoy or lack acting freely and of their own free will) and insofar as a person's agential desires will not be peculiar to her *qua* person, it will be argued in the next chapter that a person can only truly identify with an effective first-order desire if it is a personal, and not merely an agential, desire.[23]

## Identification is Not Necessary for Autonomy

With this brief account of what it is for a person to identify with her effective first-order desires in place, it can be shown that not only does a person's identification with an effective first-order desire fail to suffice for her also be to autonomous with respect to it but it is not necessary for this, either. It was noted previously that a person will only identify with her personal desires, and not her agential desires. This is because (as will be argued further in the next chapter) the question of whether a person acts freely and of her own free will is the question of whether she relates to her effective first-order desire in the appropriate way *qua* person, rather than *qua* agent. The property of identification is thus a property that persons can possess with respect to their desires. By contrast, however (as will be argued next), the property of autonomy is a property that persons can possess primarily with respect to their decisions—and only derivatively with respect to their effective first-order desires. That is, a person can be said to be autonomous with respect to her effective first-order desires if they are those that she is moved to act by as a result of a decision that she was autonomous with respect to.

Since this is so, then, provided that a person is autonomous with respect to the choice or decision that led to her being moved by an effective first-order desire she can be said to be autonomous with respect to that desire, *irrespective* of whether it is an agential desire or a personal desire. The question of whether a person is autonomous with respect to a particular desire is not settled by reference to the relationship that desire in question holds with respect to the objects of the other elements of her motivational-set but by reference to the decision-making process that led her to be moved by it. As such, unlike the question of whether a person acts freely and of her own free will, the question of whether a person is autonomous with respect to her effective first-order desire does not depend at all upon the status that that desire holds within her motivational taxonomy (i.e., as a personal or a merely agential desire). It is possible, then, that a person could be autonomous with respect to an effective first-order desire (i.e., she is moved to act on it because she endorsed it through a decision that she was autonomous with respect to) even though she does not identify with it (i.e., it is an agential desire). Thus, since it is possible for a person to be autonomous with respect to her effective first-order desires and yet not identify with them, a person's identification with a desire is not necessary for her to be autonomous with respect to it.

## WHY IDENTIFICATION AND AUTONOMY SHOULD NOT BE CONFLATED

The first reason why the distinct concepts of identification and autonomy should not be conflated is, of course, the most obvious: that to do so would be conceptually inaccurate, and that this is bad in itself. However, in addition to this reason why these two concepts should not be conflated there are two other, equally pressing, reasons as to why they should be kept separate.

### Desires and Decisions

The first of these two additional reasons as to why the concepts of identification and autonomy should not be conflated is similar to that just outlined: that to fail to recognize that they are distinct concepts will lead one into conceptual inaccuracy. However, this is not just to say that to conflate these concepts would be inaccurate. Rather, this reason has to do with the question of what identification and autonomy are properties of persons with respect to. By definition, identification is a property that persons possess (or lack) with respect to their effective first-order desires. Yet autonomy is not a property that persons primarily possess or lack with respect to their effective first-order desires—and this is certainly not definitionally true. The phenomena that are commonly taken to adversely affect a person's exercise of her autonomy—such as the successful exercise of interpersonal manipulation, deception, and coercion—do so through affecting the nature of the decisions that are made by the person whose autonomy they adversely affect. A physician who successfully manipulates his patients into taking a certain drug compromises their autonomy through substituting his judgment for theirs, insofar as it was he, and not they, who thus determines which drugs they take.[24] The question of whether a person is autonomous is thus primarily a question of whether she is autonomous with respect to her decisions.

Recognizing that autonomy is primarily a property of persons with respect to their decisions (and, hence, only derivatively a property of persons with respect to their effective first-order desires) is important in two ways. First, it is useful to note this simply for the sake of conceptual accuracy. Second, that autonomy is primarily a property of persons with respect to their decisions undermines the effectiveness of counterexamples based on the possibility of the invasive manipulation of a person's mental states that have been developed against various extant theories of autonomy.[25] As was discussed earlier in this volume persons are necessarily active with respect to their decisions, for decisions must be made; they do not simply come over persons, as an emotion might. As such, even if a person makes a decision on the basis of an inculcated desire she will not be passive with respect to it in the way that the proponents of such counterexamples believe. Thus, once it is recognized that autonomy is primarily a property of persons with respect to their decisions, counterexamples based on the invasive inculcation of desires will fail. And this is because they are only effective against analyses of autonomy whose proponents fail to recognize that autonomy is a property of persons with respect to mental states that they are necessarily active with respect to.

## The Importance of Autonomy in Bioethics

Recognizing that identification and autonomy are distinct concepts is also important if autonomy is to continue to retain its importance as the preeminent concept in contemporary bioethics. Autonomy's status as the preeminent concept in bioethics has recently been subject to the challenge that its judgmental relevance to debates in bioethics is unclear. Nomy Arpaly, for example, has expressed doubt that what she terms "complex autonomy theories," or CATs (i.e., those theories of autonomy that "have not been derived to deal with intuitions about moral responsibility and so cannot easily dispense with the expression 'autonomous action' and replace it with 'action for which we are morally responsible'. . .").[26] are relevant in discussions of applied ethics.[27] In particular, Arpaly holds that complex autonomy theories fail to be judgmentally relevant in discussions of bioethics, for, she believes, the criteria that are standardly used in medical practice to assess whether a person is sufficiently competent to be free from paternalistic intervention are unrelated to those that are offered by autonomy theorists to determine whether a person is autonomous with respect to her decisions (or other mental states). To support her point Arpaly quotes the criteria from *The Field Guide to Psychiatric Assessment and Treatment,* which must be met for "a person in need of medical treatment—whether psychiatric or otherwise— . . . [to] . . . be regarded as competent for the purpose of medical decision-making."[28] According to the authors of this *Field Guide*, a person must be able to understand the facts that are relevant to her medical condition, appreciate how they are relevant to her own situation, "rationally manipulate the information to arrive at a choice," and be able "to communicate that choice."[29] Arpaly then notes that "there is nothing in the guidelines about hierarchies of mental states, alienation, a subjective sense of passivity or activity, mental conflict, or wholeheartedness"—criteria that all appear in what Arpaly takes to be extant complex autonomy theories.[30] This being so, she concludes that since these guidelines have "no self-explanatory connection" to extant complex autonomy theories it is not obvious that the concept of autonomy is important to discussions in medical ethics.[31]

Arpaly is correct to hold that the class "of autonomous actions defined by CATs appear much smaller than the class of actions that, say, a patient has the right to perform without paternalistic intervention. . ."[32] However, she is mistaken to hold this view on the grounds that autonomy theory is not obviously relevant to bioethics. This is because Arpaly's suspicion that the concept of autonomy is not relevant to discussions of medical ethics is based on conflating the criteria required for a person to *identify with* her effective first-order desires with that which is required for her to be *autonomous with respect to* her decisions.[33] Arpaly rests her suspicions concerning the worth of autonomy theory for medical ethics in particular (and applied ethics in general) on the recognition that the question of whether a person is competent enough to be free from paternalistic intervention is not to be decided by reference to "hierarchies of mental states, alienation, a subjective sense of passivity or activity, mental conflict, or wholeheartedness," according to the authors of *The Field Guide to Psychiatric Assessment and Treatment*. However, once it is recognized that identification and autonomy are distinct concepts, and that the criteria that Arpaly lists have been offered as part of various analyses of *identification*, and *not* as part of various analyses of *autonomy*, it is clear that her suspicions concerning the importance of autonomy in applied ethics are not as well-founded as she believes. Even though discussions in medical practice of when a person's decisions are his own in a morally important sense might not parallel those philosophical discussions in which the criteria that Arpaly outlines play a role, these criteria do not pertain to analyses of *autonomy* but to analyses of *identification*.[34] As such, their absence in the debates over issues in both bioethics in particular and applied ethics in general does not indicate that autonomy is not relevant to these latter discussions. Of course, noting this implication of the distinction between identification and autonomy does not show that the concept of autonomy *should* play the central role that it currently enjoys in many debates within applied ethics. Arpaly is right that "Substantial argument seems required here."[35] But it does show that one should not be suspicious of the importance of *autonomy* theory for debates within applied ethics on the grounds that Arpaly outlines.[36]

## OBJECTIONS

The view that identification and autonomy are distinct concepts, and that it is theoretically important for discussions of both to recognize this, is a novel one, and so is unlikely to gain ready acceptance, either by persons who take themselves primarily to be theorists of identification, or of autonomy. As such, it is going to be faced with numerous objections. Although some of these have already been addressed in Chapter 1, where the account of practical autonomy that is the mainstay of this volume was developed and defended, and some will be addressed in the discussion of identification in the next chapter, two initial objections to the claim that the concepts of identification and autonomy should be addressed now.

### An Exegetical Objection

The first of these initial objections is an exegetical one. Although Frankfurt does not mention autonomy in his early papers, as Paul Benson observes the metaphors that he uses to outline the connotative contours of the concept that he is analyzing "are among the most vivid and compelling" that have been offered. Furthermore, as Benson notes, these metaphors are apt ones to capture the connotative contours of the concept of autonomy: "A person who acts autonomously genuinely 'participates' in the operation of her will, as opposed to being 'estranged' from herself or being a 'helpless or passive bystander to the forces that move' her. Agents who act intentionally but without autonomy do not do what they 'really want' to do; their effective volitions are 'external to' or 'outside' them."[37] As such, even though Frankfurt did not explicitly mention the concept of autonomy in his early work on identification, it seems appropriate to hold that these concepts are coextensive. Moreover, this first exegetical objection to the previous argument in favor of distinguishing these concepts is not based merely upon the aptness of Frankfurt's metaphors for both the concepts of identification and autonomy: there is also reason to think that he intends to offer his hierarchical analysis of identification as an analysis of autonomy. For example, in "Autonomy, Necessity, and Love," Frankfurt claimed that "The distinction between heteronomy and autonomy coincides. . .with the distinction between being passive and being active."[38] This makes it plausible to believe that, for Frankfurt, for a person to identify with her effective first-order desires is also for her to be autonomous with respect to them.[39]

Yet although this exegetical objection to the prior argument in favor of distinguishing between identification and autonomy is plausible, there are three good reasons to reject it. First, the mere fact that Frankfurt's metaphors are apt for both autonomy and identification does not show that these concepts are coextensive; it just shows that they have similar connotations. And this should not be surprising in the context of this discussion, for were the connotations of these concepts not to be similar they would never have been conflated. Second, although Frankfurt wrote in "Autonomy, Necessity, and Love" that he was interested in that essay "in autonomy," he addresses two distinct (albeit related) issues in it.[40] In the first part of "Autonomy, Necessity, and Love" he addresses the differences between his conception of personal autonomy, whereby a "person acts autonomously only when his volitions derive from the essential character of his will," and Kant's impersonal conception of autonomy, on which the autonomous will "must conform. . .to the requirements of a will that is indifferent to all personal interests."[41] In the second part of this essay, however, Frankfurt does not mention autonomy at all. Instead, he addresses the relationships that hold between a personal identity, loving something, and identifying with those effective first-order desires that spring from one's loving something. To be sure, these two separate discussions in this essay are clearly related to each other. However, that they are clearly separated within this essay serves to undercut the previous exegetical objection to distinguishing identification and autonomy in the way argued for previously, for this separation indicates that there is a distinction to be drawn between the concepts of autonomy and identification. Finally, and most importantly, the prior objection to distinguishing between identification and autonomy suffers from a serious lacuna. That a person must be active with respect to his effective first-order desires to identify with them, and must also be active with respect to his decisions (and the desires and actions that flow from them) to be autonomous with respect to them, does *not* show that a person's identification with his effective first-order desires is either necessary or sufficient for him to be autonomous with respect to them. That X is necessary for both P and Q does not show that P and Q are coextensive concepts.

## Identification and Autonomy are Differing Conceptions of the Same Concept

The second initial objection to distinguishing between the concepts of identification and autonomy is similar to the first, in that it is based upon the fact that the connotations of identification and autonomy are very similar.

Drawing on this recognition, one might argue that even though there might be significant differences between the denotations of identification and of autonomy, as outlined previously, these differences are not significant enough to justify the claim that these are distinct concepts. Rather, the proponent of this objection could claim, identification and autonomy are simply two differing conceptions of the same concept, and that it is immaterial as to whether this overarching concept is termed "identification" or "autonomy."

There are, however, three main reasons as to why this second objection to distinguishing between autonomy and identification is misplaced. The first of these reasons is simply methodological. As was noted in the Introduction to this volume given the numerous ways in which the term "autonomy" is used it behooves anyone who utilizes this concept to state explicitly what its denotations are being taken to be. As such, rather than moving to using this concept less precisely (as would be the result of accepting this second objection) one should instead strive to use it more precisely. Secondly, and more importantly, since a person's identification with one of her effective first-order desires is neither necessary nor sufficient for her to be (derivatively) autonomous with respect to it, it is clear that "identification" and "autonomy" are *not* merely differing conceptions of the same concept. Finally, this point is reinforced by the recognition that, as was argued in Chapter 1, autonomy is a political concept, and, as will be further argued in the next chapter, identification is a metaphysical concept, and so discussions of them should take place within two different arenas of philosophical debate.


CONCLUSION

It has been argued in this chapter that identification and autonomy are distinct concepts and that a person's identification with her effective first-order desires is neither necessary nor sufficient for her to be autonomous with respect to them. Distinguishing between identification and autonomy is thus an important step to take to provide an adequate account of either— just as the development of such accounts are necessary to show that these are indeed distinct concepts. This distinction between identification and autonomy is not, however, merely a theoretical nicety. Not only does it clarify these concepts and thus aid the achievement of conceptual accuracy, but it also serves to show that certain criticisms of the centrality of autonomy in contemporary bioethics are misguided, for they are based upon conflating this concept with that of identification. To buttress these points, an account of identification will be developed and defended in the next chapter. This account will not only be firmly positioned within the mainstream discussion of this concept but will also be developed in such a way as to make clear its metaphysical, rather than political, orientation. As such, the aim of the next chapter is not only to develop a theoretically satisfying account of identification that is distinct from that of autonomy but also to show how this concept is not relevant to those debates within bioethics in which the latter concept plays a central role. In so doing a far, far better account of these concepts will be provided than has ever been done before.[42]

# 4 Decisive Identification

In Chapter 1 an account of autonomy was developed and defended—
"practical autonomy"—that captured the connotative contours of this
concept as it is used in contemporary philosophical discussion. With this
account in hand, it was argued in Chapter 2 that there was good reason
to adopt this account of practical autonomy as a (if not *the*) core account
of this concept, since there were fewer faces of autonomy than it might, at
first, appear. Then, in Chapter 3, it was argued that the concepts of autonomy and identification are distinct, with the former, and not the latter,
being that which enjoys prominence in contemporary bioethics. Given the
arguments of these three chapters, then, it might appear that a discussion of
the metaphysical question of the conditions that must be met for a person
to identify with her effective first-order desires would be out of place in a
volume devoted to developing an account of autonomy for use in contemporary moral philosophy, in general, and bioethics, in particular. But this
appearance is misleading, for two reasons. First, for the arguments in the
previous chapter to be fully convincing, an account of identification must
be provided to show that autonomy and identification really *are* distinct
concepts—and that it is the former, and not the latter, that is the dominant
concept of contemporary bioethics. Second (and relatedly) as was noted in
both Chapters 2 and 3 the concept of identification is often conflated with
that of autonomy. Offering an analysis of identification would thus be useful for bioethicists, insofar as this would underscore the point that this is
a metaphysical concept, and not a political one—and thus not one that is
immediately germane to many of their discussions.

Since the publication of Harry Frankfurt's seminal paper "Freedom of the
Will and the Concept of a Person" there has been no shortage of attempts to
provide an analysis of identification (even if some of those attempting this
believed that they were providing an analysis of autonomy). It has become
common for persons who attempt such an analysis first to outline the three
standard problems that are held to beset Frankfurt's original account of
identification (the *Ab Initio* Problem, the Problem of Manipulation, and

the Regress-cum- Incompleteness Problem), and then, with these problems in hand, attempt to provide an analysis of identification that avoids them all.[1] The approach taken in this chapter will, however, differ from this. Instead of simply outlining these problems as they appear in the literature, each of them will be assessed to determine if it is a genuine problem that must be addressed in developing an account of identification, or if it is only a pseudo-problem in that context, whose force is drawn from conflating intuitions about identification with intuitions about autonomy. Once the genuine problems for analyses of identification have been recognized and the requirements that they impose upon analyses of identification in order for them to be avoided have been identified, the conditions that must be met for a person to identify with her effective first-order desires will be outlined. With these in hand, it will be clear that a person's identification with her effective first-order desires will neither be necessary nor sufficient for her to be autonomous with respect to them.

## APPARENT PROBLEMS FOR FRANKFURT'S
## ORIGINAL ANALYSIS OF IDENTIFICATION

In "Freedom of the Will and the Concept of a Person" Frankfurt is concerned with three related questions: the "problem of understanding what it is to be a creature that not only has a mind and a body but is also a person,"[2] the question of "what kind of freedom is the freedom of the will,"[3] and the question of when a person "is morally responsible for what he has done."[4] Frankfurt considers that what is essential to an individual's being a person is that he have what he terms "'second-order volitions' or 'volitions of the second order.'"[5] That is, for Frankfurt, it is essential for an individual to be a person that he not only have first-order desires (e.g., "I want to smoke") and desires about those desires (e.g., "I want to want to smoke"), but that he have desires about which of his first-order desires be effective in moving him to act. With this in hand, Frankfurt argues that a person will enjoy freedom of the will when "he is free to will what he wants to will, or to have the will he wants," and so "It is securing the conformity of his will to his second-order volitions. . .that a person exercises freedom of the will."[6] However, a person need not, argues Frankfurt, enjoy freedom of the will to be morally responsible for his actions. Instead, a person could be morally responsible for an act if he performed it "freely, or that he did it of his own free will," that he was moved to act by a will that he wanted to be moved by, whether or not this will was under his control.[7] All three of the previous questions, then, turn on the issue of whether the individual at issue in each of them is capable of identifying with his effective first-order desires, or has identified himself with the effective first-order desire that moved him to perform the act in question, where such identification is constituted, for Frankfurt, "through the formation of a second-order volition."[8]

In "Freedom of the Will and the Concept of a Person" Frankfurt held that a person identifies with his effective first-order desires if he both wants to have them and wants them to move him to act. This initial analysis of identification, however, has been held to be subject to three serious objections.[9] The first of these is the *Ab Initio* Problem (also termed the Problem of Authority). In holding that a person will act freely and of her own free will in when she endorses her effective first-order desire with a second-order volition Frankfurt is according authority to a person's second-order volitions that is not possessed by her first-order desires. But a person's second-order volitions are themselves simply a type of desire.[10] As such, how does the mere fact that a person endorses her effective first-order desires with them ensure that such endorsed desires are more truly her own? The second problem that Frankfurt's original account of identification is held to face is the Problem of Manipulation. Frankfurt's original account of identification was a structural account, on which a person will identify with his effective first-order desires if they possess certain structural relationships to other aspects of his preference structure. As such, it appears that Frankfurt is committed to holding that a person will identify with an effective first-order desire even if both it and his volitional endorsement of it were implanted into him by, for example, a nefarious neurosurgeon. However, since such an implanted desire seems to be one that is paradigmatically alien to the person into whom it has been implanted, such examples seem to serve as counterexamples to Frankfurt's initial analysis of identification.[11] The final major problem that Frankfurt's account of identification is held to be subject to is the Regress-cum-Incompleteness Problem. As Gary Watson has urged, "Since second-order volitions are themselves simply desires, to add them to the context of conflict is just to increase the number of contenders; it is not to give special place to any of those in contention."[12] Since this is so, it will be an open question as to whether the person whose effective first-order desires are at issue identifies with his relevant second-order volitions. If the answer is that he does because he has a higher-order volition that endorses them, then the question will simply reappear at this level of volition. This is the Regress Problem. If, however, the answer is that he is because he identifies with his second-order volitions in a manner that is different from how he identifies with his effective first-order desires, then the account of identification that Frankfurt initially offered was incomplete. This is the Incompleteness Problem.

## RESPONDING TO THE PROBLEMS

Yet although these three problems are standardly held to beset Frankfurt's initial account of identification not all of them are applicable to it. The *Ab Initio* Problem was first developed against Frankfurt's account of identification by John Christman, who explicitly understood Frankfurt's account of what it is for a person to identify with her desires to be synonymous with what it is for her to be autonomous with respect to them.[13] Christman held that the *Ab Initio* Problem was a problem for Frankfurt's view insofar as Frankfurt's account of identification implied that "a person can have autonomous first-order desires despite having nonautonomous higher-order desires." That is, it implied that a person could fail to identify with her second-order volitions (as Frankfurt offered no account of how a person would necessarily identify with them) and yet still be autonomous with respect to her effective first-order desires that were endorsed by them. If Frankfurt's account of what it is for a person to identify with her effective first-order desires was indeed an account of what it is for her to be autonomous with respect to them it is clear how this would (at least on the face of it) be a problem for his view. An autonomous person is supposed to be "under his or her own control, master of his or her own destiny."[14] As such, then, if a person does not have control over her higher-order volitions, and so, apparently, is not autonomous with respect to them, it would seem that she cannot be autonomous with respect to those of her effective first-order desires that such uncontrolled volitions endorse. The lack of control that she is subject to at her higher conative level would flow down to her lower-order desires. Whether this version of the *Ab Initio* Problem (i.e., that which is aimed at conceptions of autonomy on which persons can be autonomous with respect to their effective first-order desires, but not with respect to other elements of their preference structure that motivated them to act on the effective first-order desires in question) is cogent or not in the context of personal autonomy will be discussed more fully in Chapter 7. Given, however, that Frankfurt is analyzing identification in the context of developing compatibilist accounts of freedom of the will and of what it is to act freely and of one's own free will it is clear that it is not a cogent objection to his view of what it is for a person to *identify with* her effective first-order desires. The *Ab Initio* objection against Frankfurt's initial account of identification is based on the assumption that to have the sort of control that is necessary for a person to identify with her effective first-order desires she must have full control over the states of affairs that led her volitionally to endorse them. But to accept this assumption would be to preclude the possibility that a compatibilist account of identification could be correct. This is because the proponents of such an account would accept that it is possible that the person whose desires are in question lives in a determined universe, and so it is possible that she would lack the sort of control that this assumption requires. As such, then, to offer the *Ab Initio* objection to Frankfurt's metaphysically compatibilist account of identification is simply to beg the question against it.[15]

Christman, then, is mistaken to hold that the *Ab Initio* Problem is a live problem for Frankfurt's account of identification. Yet although the *Ab Initio* Problem is not relevant to Frankfurt's original account of identification the same cannot be said of either the Problem of Manipulation or the

Regress-cum-Incompleteness Problem. The Problem of Manipulation shows that any adequate account of identification must incorporate a historical component: it must require that a person's identification with a desire came about in a certain way—or at least that it did not come about in certain ways (e.g., through implantation). The Regress-cum-Incompleteness Problem shows that the type of historical process that the desires that a person identifies with must have arisen from (or be precluded from arising from) must be an objective, rather than a subjective, process. That is to say, it must be a process that requires that a desire meet certain objective criteria as a necessary condition of the person whose desire it is identifying with it. It cannot be the case that the historical criteria that are required are purely subjective, for then it will also be an open question as to whether or not the person in question identifies with her attitudes of endorsement—and this will lead straight back to the Regress-cum-Incompleteness Problem.[16] As such, the historical process from which desires that persons can be legitimately held to identify with must be one with respect to which the question of whether a person could fail to identify with a desire that was produced by it cannot arise. Finally, even though the historical process from which the desires that a person can correctly be said to identify with must be an objective one, it cannot be the case that the subjective attitude of the person whose desires they are is eliminated altogether from the process that leads to her identifying with them. If the conditions that must be met for an individual to identify with her effective first-order desires were purely objective conditions (e.g., they must arise in the right way from her basic desires with respect to which she must be identified) then there is a possibility that they could be met by nonpersons. If, for example, it was held that an individual would identify with her effective first-order desires if they nondeviantly arose from that subset of her preferences with respect to which the question of whether or not they are truly hers cannot arise, it could be the case that a nonperson with the appropriate preference structure could be held to identify with its desires. And this possibility must be precluded, for an account of what it is for a person to identify with her effective first-order desires should also be an account of what it is for an agent to act freely and of his own free will—and these are attributes only of persons. To preclude this possibility, then, any satisfactory account of identification will have to follow Frankfurt's lead and require that the individual whose desires are in question adopt a reflexive attitude towards them of a sort that only persons could hold.

## WHAT'S PAST IS PROLOGUE

For a person to identify with her effective first-order desires, then, they must meet two conditions: (i) they must be the result of a process with respect to which the question of whether their possessor would fail to identify with desires produced by it cannot arise, and (ii) their possessor must adopt a reflexive attitude of endorsement towards them that only a person can adopt.[17] There are two approaches that could be taken to develop an analysis of identification that would meet this pair of conditions. First, one could attempt to develop a *structural* account of identification. Focusing on condition (i), the proponent of such an approach to analyzing identification would attempt to identify a way in which first-order desires could be produced that would preclude the possibility of their possessor's failing to identify with them. The proponent of such an approach might, for example, hold that there is a subset of desires within persons' preference systems from which they cannot be alienated, because they are fully or partially constitutive of their selves. With this in hand she would then argue that provided that a person's effective first-order desires flowed from this subset in a way that would preclude her from being alienated from them they would meet condition (i). One way in which a person's effective first-order desires could flow from her subset of inalienable desires would be if they were produced by a combination of an inalienable desire and a belief that she had accepted after subjecting it to critical assessment. An implanted desire would not satisfy this condition, since such a desire would not have been produced by a belief–desire pair such that the belief in question was one that the person into whom the desire had been implanted had accepted after subjecting it to critical reflection.[18] Were a person's effective first-order desire not to have been produced directly by a belief–*inalienable desire* pair, then she could identify with it on this account were it to have been produced by a belief–desire pair where the desire in question was generated directly by an earlier belief–inalienable desire pair, or indirectly, in that it was the product of a string of belief–desire pairs that were grounded in a belief–inalienable desire pair.[19] Since such a structural account of identification requires a person to critically reflect upon the beliefs that, in combination with desires, motivate a person to have her effective first-order desires, it will also satisfy condition (ii), for it would be held that such reflection is the province only of persons.[20] Alternatively, one could attempt to develop an *attitudinal* account of identification. Focusing on condition (ii), the proponent of such an account of identification will hold that a person will identify with her effective first-order desires if she endorses them with an attitude that is not only one that only persons could adopt but which is one with respect to which the question of whether she is alienated from it could not arise. The endorsement of an effective first-order desire by such an attitude would thus constitute a person's identification with it.

The prior structural approach to analyzing identification faces an obvious difficulty. To ground an account of identification on a subset of a person's preference system from which she cannot be alienated as it is (at least partially) constitutive of who she is, is to ground an account of identification on an account of personal identity.[21] And, since developing an account of personal identity is at least as difficult as developing an account of identification, the proponents of such an approach to this problem seem to be moving out of the frying pan and into the fire.[22] This difficulty that is faced by the proponents of the structural approach to analyzing identification is, however, avoidable, for a fully satisfactory attitudinal analysis of identification can be developed from Frankfurt's work on decisive identification.

Recognizing the difficulty that was posed to his initial account of identification by the Regress-cum-Incompleteness Problem Frankfurt held that

> When a person identifies himself decisively with one of his first-order desires, this commitment "resounds" throughout the potentially endless array of higher orders. Consider a person who, without reservation or conflict, wants to be motivated by the desire to concentrate on his work. The fact that his second-order volition to be moved by this desire is a decisive one means that there is no room for questions concerning the pertinence of desires or volitions of higher orders. Suppose the person is asked whether he wants to want to want to concentrate on his work. He can properly insist that this question concerning a third-order desire does not arise.[23]

Frankfurt elaborated this account of decisive identification in a later essay, acknowledging that the "notions" that he drew upon in the quoted passage ("'identification,' 'decisive commitment,' 'resounding'") were "terribly obscure."[24] Responding to Watson's charge that any such decision to identify oneself with an effective first-order desire would simply be arbitrary,[25] Frankfurt compared the situation of a person who was wondering whether to identify himself with one of his effective first-order desires to that a person attempting to solve an arithmetical problem.[26] Noting both that a person might indefinitely check his calculations to ensure that they are correct, and that there is nothing special about any one such check that would give it authority over the others solely by virtue of its location within the sequences of checks, Frankfurt observed that a person could cease to check his calculations once he has decided for a reason to adopt a certain result. He might, for example, believe that his result is correct, and so further checking would be pointless, or he might believe that although there is some possibility that it is in error the cost to him of checking further would outweigh the possible benefits that he might gain from this. Once a person has decided to stop checking his calculations, then, no matter what reason led him to decide this, he could be sure that *that* decision would be one that he would always reaffirm were he to revisit it. Such a person's checking of his arithmetic is analogous, claims Frankfurt, to a person's questioning whether he wants to want a certain first-order desire to be his will; whether he wants to want to satisfy a certain desire, and for it thus to move him to act. Just as a person might nonarbitrarily decide to terminate his checking of his calculations, then, so too might a person nonarbitrarily decide to cease examining his desires to see if they are the ones who he really wants to be moved by. And when a person does so, he will *decisively identify with* the desires by which he wishes to be moved.[27]

It is important to note that whereas such decisive identification is necessary for a person to identify with a desire, as will be argued next it is not sufficient, and so Frankfurt's account of decisive identification needs to be supplemented with a further condition. Before moving to argue for this latter claim it should be noted that this account of decisive identification meets both condition (i) and condition (ii)—although Frankfurt did not recognize this. In deciding that a particular desire is a desire by which he wishes to be moved an agent will be adopting an attitude towards it that only a person could adopt, for only persons assess the desirability of their desires in this way. As such, the decisive identification component of this account of identification satisfies condition (ii). It also satisfies condition (i). A person is necessarily active with respect to the decisions that he makes; it is impossible for a person to be passive with respect to them. Persons *make* decisions; they do not "come over them," as emotions can. A person, then, cannot be alienated from her decisions. As such, if a person decides to identify with a particular first-order desire, there is no room for the question of whether or not such an identification is really hers to arise—and so condition (i) is satisfied.[28]

That a person *decisively identifies* with an effective first-order desire is necessary for her to identify (simpliciter) with it, but it is not sufficient for this. To see this, consider Frankfurt's examples of the unwilling and the willing addicts.[29] The unwilling addict "hates his addiction and always struggles desperately, although to no avail, against its thrust. He tries everything that he thinks might enable him to overcome his desires for the drug. But these desires are too powerful for him to withstand, and invariably, in the end, they conquer him."[30] By contrast, although the willing addict's addiction "has the same physiological basis and the same irresistible thrust as the additions of the unwilling addict . . . he is altogether delighted with his condition . . . [he] would not have things any other way . . . "[31] When the willing addict takes the drug to which he is addicted he does so freely and of his own free will, whereas the unwilling addict does not. This difference between the addicts cannot be explained by claiming that whereas the willing addict decisively identifies with his effective first-order desire the unwilling addict does not. This is because in implicitly assuming that the unwilling addicted is completely passive with respect to the satisfaction of his desire for the drug this explanation misdescribes his motivational structure. This addict is not simply reduced to the status of an automaton when his desire for the drug moves him to act. Instead, even though he will invariably succumb to its thrust, he decides when this will be, by deciding when he will no longer tolerate the pain that resisting it causes him. Unlike the willing addict, then, the unwilling addict is not directly motivated by his desire for the drug; his actions are not performed to satisfy the desire whose object is to take the drug. Rather, he is indirectly motivated by this desire, in that resisting it causes pain, and so he takes the drug to satisfy his desire to avoid pain.[32] The unwilling addict, then, *does* decisively identify with the desire that moves him to take the drug to which he is addicted (i.e., the desire to avoid pain). How, then, is he to be differentiated form the willing addict? The answer to this question lies in the type of desire that each addict acts to satisfy. The willing addict acts to satisfy a desire that is not shared by all normally constituted agents (i.e., for the drug) whereas the desire that the unwilling addict acts to satisfy is (i.e., to avoid pain). The unwilling addict, then, does not act freely and of his own free will when he takes the drug to which he is addicted because he is motivated to act by an *agential* desire, a desire that is held in common by all normally constituted agents. When a person acts on an agential desire he will not be acting qua person but qua agent—and this is so even if he reflexively endorses his being moved by the desire in question in a manner that is only available to persons. Since the ability to act freely and of their own free wills is an ability that only persons can have or lack, when a person acts qua agent (that is, when he acts to satisfy an agential desire), the question of whether or not he acts freely and of his own free will is inapplicable to him. Thus, for a person to identify with his effective first-order desires he must not only decisively identify himself with them, but they must be nonagential desires; that is, they must be desires that are not shared with all other normally constituted agents.[33]

## OBJECTIONS AND REPLIES

Although as was noted at the start of this chapter the previous account of what it is for a person to identify with her effective first-order is only an outline of how such identification is to be understood it is still subject to three immediate objections.

### Velleman's Objection

The first objection to the previous account of identification is a reiteration of one that has been discussed already, in the context of its being leveled against the account of autonomy that was developed in Chapter 1. This objection is that which could be drawn from Velleman's discussion of apparently passive decisions: that, like emotions, decisions can simply come over people in such a way that they are not active with respect to them.[34] If persons can be passive with respect to their decisions in this way, then the question can be raised of whether or not a person could fail to identify with the decisions that he makes—and if this is so then the account of decisive identification that was developed previously will fail to meet condition (i). As was discussed in Chapter 1, however, this objection will not work, for Velleman's description of how a decision motivates a person to act is phenomenologically inaccurate. Decisions do not simply come over one in this way; it is necessary that a decision be made, and the making of a decision necessarily requires that the agent whose decision it is be actively involved in this. It is thus simply not true that decisions can be "induced in me but not formed by me," as Velleman claims.[35]

## A Further Problem of Manipulation

The claim that a person can be passive with respect to her decisions, and thus that the previous account of decisive identification will fail to meet condition (i), can, however, be supported in another way. The prior attitudinal account of decisive identification places no restrictions upon the reasons that could lead a person to decide to identify with a particular first-order desire of hers. As such, it is possible that a person might be manipulated into making a particular decision by another person. Consider, for example, a person who has certain desires hypnotically induced into her by another who does so in order to lead her to make a certain decision, and, as a result of these desires, the manipulee is led to make the decision that her manipulator wants her to make. Surely in this case, one might argue, the person who is subject to such manipulation is passive with respect to her decision-making process? And, if this is so, then the account of decisive identification that was outlined will fail to meet condition (i).[36]

Yet although, as was argued in Chapter 1, being subject to such manipulation would render a person nonautonomous with respect to her decisions and the effective first-order desires and actions that flow from them, it would not undermine a person's identification with the desires that she thus came to decisively identify with. Unlike the concept of autonomy, there is nothing in the concept of identification that precludes a person from acting freely and of her own free will even when the ultimate explanation for her making the decisions that she does lies in the will of another agent. Since this is so, the person who is subject to such manipulation will still be active with respect to her decision in the relevant sense for her to act freely and of her own free will, for it will still be *she* who makes it, even if she does so at the behest of another. As Frankfurt puts it, when a person subject to such manipulation "provides the passion with meaning, or somehow construes it as having a natural place in his experience . . . [then . . . despite its origin, the passion becomes attached to a moving principle within the person; and the person is no more a passive bystander with respect to it than if it had arisen in more integral response to his perceptions."[37] Like the original Problem of Manipulation, then, this version of it can also be avoided by the previous account of decisive identification.

## Not All Actions are Performed Decisively

The final objection that this account of decisive identification is initially beset by is simple: that it seems severe to restrict the number of actions that persons perform freely and of their own free will. An example that has been developed by David Pears demonstrates this point well: "a man walking along a beach sees what may be the keel of a surfboard or a dead fish and curiosity leads him to go and find out which it is. He does it just because he feels like it."[38] This man did not decide to look at the object on the beach; he just did so because he felt like doing so. As such, then, it seems that he did not do so freely and of his own free will if the prior account of decisive identification is to be accepted—and at first sight this seems implausible.

This objection, however, can be readily met. The claim that the conclusion that the man in Pears's example did not move to look at the object on the beach freely and of his own free will is implausible gains its force from the idea that if a person did not do something freely and of his own free will then it is not attributable to him. But this restriction on the attributability of actions to agents is not an implication of this account of identification, for on this account of identification actions can still be attributed to persons qua agents. Moreover, given that persons are (counterfactually) capable of decisively performing those actions that are theirs qua agents (i.e., they could have performed them after deciding to do so in the appropriate way, even if they performed them without decisively identifying with them), then they could still be held to be morally responsible for them.[39] Indeed, that this account of identification does not hold that all actions attributable to persons are those that they perform freely and of their own free will is a strength of this analysis, not a weakness. It provides a richer and more accurate taxonomy of desires and actions than the usual binary distinction between those desires that a person identifies with (and those actions that she thus performs freely and of her own free will), and those that she is alienated from.[40] This is because it allows persons to have desires and actions attributed to them (i.e., in their capacity as agents) without committing the ascriber to holding that the persons in question identify with the desires in question, or performed the acts freely and of their own free will.

## CONCLUSION

With both this account of decisive identification and the account of autonomy that was developed in Chapter 1 in place, then, the conclusion of the previous chapter is reinforced: that a person's identification with her effective first-order desires is neither necessary nor sufficient for her to be (derivatively) autonomous with respect to them. Moreover, since identification is an *internalist* concept (that is, the question of whether or not a person identifies with any one of her effective first-order desires can be answered by reference to her mental states alone) it is clear that it is not relevant to the bioethical issues in which the *externalist* concept of autonomy plays a central role. The nature of the relationships that a person has with others is irrelevant to the question of whether or not she identifies with those of her effective first-order desires that she forms as a result of them. For example, as was shown by the example of Othello and Iago in the previous chapter, a person could fully identify with her first-order desires even if she possesses them as a result of being unwittingly subject to the deception or manipulation of others. Given this, then, the concept of identification is not relevant to those debates in bioethics in which the concept of autonomy plays a central role, for these debates are typically concerned with assessing whether certain ways of treating persons either fail to respect the autonomy of persons, or else adversely affect it. As such, then, recognizing the distinction between the concepts of identification and autonomy, and then, with this in hand, expressly focusing on the latter is a consummation devoutly to be wished for all areas of moral philosophy, in general, and bioethics in particular, in whose discussions autonomy plays a central role.

# 5   Autonomy and Normativity

## INTRODUCTION

Thus far in this volume an account of practical autonomy has been developed and defended (in Chapter 1), and, with this in hand, it was established in Chapter 2 that the concept of autonomy is not as hydra-headed as it might at first appear. It was then argued in Chapter 3 that autonomy and identification are distinct concepts, which laid the groundwork for the development (in Chapter 4) of an account of decisive identification. With this theoretical background in place it is time now to turn to develop further this account of practical autonomy through showing how a person's autonomy is affected by an increase in the number of options from which she has to choose and how it is affected by her being subject to constraints. These discussions of the effects that increased choice and constraint have upon the autonomy of those faced with, or subjected to, them will not, however, be merely theoretically orientated. Instead, they will be developed so that they illuminate not only the theory of practical autonomy that is the focus of this volume but also those debates in biomedical ethics that turn on the relationships that hold between autonomy, choice, and constraint.

## BIOETHICS AND CONTENT-NEUTRAL AUTONOMY

Before turning to discuss the relationships that hold between this account of practical autonomy, and choice and constraint, and from this to shed light on debates in bioethics in which these relationships play a central role, it is necessary to consider one of the features of practical autonomy that appears to be one of its major strengths qua an account of autonomy that has been developed to play the central role that has been accorded to this concept in contemporary bioethics. Considering this apparent feature of practical autonomy is necessary not only to emphasize how appropriate this account of autonomy is for contemporary bioethics but also because this appropriateness arises from an aspect of this account of practical autonomy that some theorists consider a significant weakness.

The feature of practical autonomy that is at issue here is its (supposed) content-neutrality, on which no restrictions are placed on the desires or values that could motivate a person to perform an action that she was autonomous with respect to. (Sigurdur Kristinsson notes that there are two types of content-neutral accounts of autonomy: procedural accounts, on which "an action is autonomous if it is motivated by a desire that has come about in the right way," and structural accounts, on which "the desire's content must fit correctly with the desires that are central to the person's character").[1] The apparent content-neutrality of this account of practical autonomy stands in contrast to substantive accounts of autonomy on which (weakly) a person cannot endorse certain values (e.g., thoroughgoing servility) if she is to be autonomous, or (strongly) her acceptance of certain values (such as that of her own autonomy) is a necessary precondition for her to be autonomous.[2] On its face the apparent content-neutrality of this account of practical autonomy is a significant strength, for it enables its proponents to recognize persons as autonomous no matter what their values might be. As such, this account of autonomy would seem to be well-suited to contemporary discussions of bioethics. This is because such discussions now take place (at least in Western liberal societies) against the background of a pluralistic culture in which the individuals involved (be they healthcare professionals, policy makers, or patients) not only might not share the same values but might even have values that conflict. Thus, to accord with the liberal ethos of the societies in which such pluralism is often found and hence to avoid the imposition of values upon persons who do not share them (and even, perhaps, who reject them) a framework for bioethical and medical decision-making should be constructed that allows persons to choose for themselves which course of action to pursue, while enabling them to seek the guidance of others should they wish to do so.[3] In this context a content-neutral account of autonomy would naturally appear to be the core value that should guide the construction of such a decision-making framework.[4] This is because, first, an emphasis on autonomy would serve as a bulwark against one person (or group of persons) imposing their values upon another.[5] Second, given that this emphasis on the value of autonomy stemmed from the recognition of values pluralism and the belief that this should be accommodated through constructing a framework for decision-making to (at best) avoid or (at worst) minimize persons having values imposed on them that they do not share, the account of autonomy that would undergird this framework should not be one that precluded certain persons from being recognized as being autonomous on the basis of their values. Given these considerations, then, the account of autonomy that should play the role that has been accorded to this concept in contemporary bioethics should, it seems, be one that is content-neutral, rather than substantive. And thus since the account of practical autonomy that was developed in Chapter 1 appears to be such an account, it appears to be well-suited to assume the role accorded to this concept in bioethics.

But this apparent strength of the account of practical autonomy that was developed in Chapter 1 might also be a weakness. In recent years content-neutral accounts of autonomy have been subject to two lines of criticism. First, they have been criticized on the grounds that they fail to recognize that the standard use of the concept of autonomy is implicitly based upon the view that to be autonomous a person must endorse certain values. Thus, since content-neutral analyses of autonomy will necessarily fail to capture the implicit normative presuppositions that undergird this concept they are inadequate. (The proponents of this objection often go on to develop substantive accounts of autonomy.) Second, they have been criticized on the grounds that it is partially constitutive of the concept of autonomy that an autonomous person must be capable of detecting and appropriately responding to certain values or reasons. (The proponents of this objection often go on to develop what can be termed "normative competence" accounts of autonomy, on which a necessary condition for a person to be autonomous with respect to her actions is that she recognize certain reasons or values as being salient to her decision-making.) Hence, since content-neutral accounts of autonomy do not impose this requirement on persons they fail to be satisfactory.

With the previous discussion of why an account of autonomy should be content-neutral to play its central role in contemporary discussions of bio-ethics in hand, it might appear that if one is interested in developing such an account of autonomy then one should defend content-neutral analyses of autonomy from the prior two criticisms. The first aim of this chapter is, however, the opposite of this: to argue that content-neutral analyses of autonomy are indeed impoverished and that a proper understanding of autonomy should lead one to endorse a substantive account of this concept. Despite appearances, however, this conclusion should not concern those who believe that a content-neutral account of autonomy is required to play the central role that it has in contemporary bioethics. The substance of the account of autonomy that these criticisms of content-neutral analyses will show is necessary for any satisfactory conception of autonomy to possess will be so thin that any account of autonomy that possessed it—including that developed in Chapter 1—could still readily play this central role. Indeed, this substance will be so thin that the previous two criticisms of content-neutral accounts of autonomy could still be leveled at the mini-mally substantive approach to autonomy that will be defended in the first part of this chapter. The proponents of the first of these criticisms will hold that this account of autonomy is too minimal and that it fails to acknowl-edge that certain values are implicit within the concept of autonomy, while the proponents of the second will hold that it still fails to acknowledge that an autonomous person must recognize and respond to certain reasons and values. The second aim of this chapter will thus be to show that these two objections that could be leveled against the minimally substantive account of autonomy developed in Chapter 1 are mistaken.

## AGAINST CONTENT-NEUTRAL ACCOUNTS OF AUTONOMY

As Kristinsson observes, "Leading accounts of personal autonomy are *content-neutral*," with their proponents insisting that "there are no a priori constraints on the content of the desires or values that might motivate an autonomous action."[6] To illustrate this claim Kristinsson notes that Dworkin holds that "the autonomous person can be a tyrant or a slave, a saint or a sinner, a rugged individualist or a champion of fraternity, a leader or a follower," and that "There is nothing in the idea of autonomy that precludes a person from saying, 'I want to be the kind of person who acts at the command of others. I define myself as a slave and endorse those attitudes and preferences. My autonomy consists in being a slave.'"[7] Similarly, Kristinsson quotes Christman's claim that "any desire, no matter how evil, self-sacrificing, or slavish it might be" could be one that its possessor was autonomous with respect to,[8] and he notes that, according to Richard Double, "not only could any desire pass the relevant procedural tests [for its possessor to be autonomous with respect to it on a content-neutral account of autonomy], but also that the tests themselves should be relative to the individual's characteristic 'style' of managing decisions."[9]

Kristinsson argues that such content-neutral accounts of autonomy fail, for they commit their proponents to holding that persons who are paradigmatically heteronomous with respect to their actions are actually autonomous with respect to them. To show this, Kristinsson draws on the example of Fatma Mint Mamadou, who has been a slave all of her life and who believes that God created her to be a slave. Fatma "has no desire to lead a life other than that of submissive obedience," and also seems "to lack basic self-respect."[10] Fatma, then, is "content to live by other people's choices"; it is thus not she, but they, who guide and direct her actions.[11] Fatma is thus paradigmatically heteronomous with respect to her actions. With this in hand, Kristinsson argues that defenders of content-neutral accounts of autonomy have the following options for dealing with the case of Fatma:

  (i) Argue that as Fatma is described, her obedient actions couldn't possibly satisfy the favored procedural or structural criteria.
 (ii) Admit that Fatma might satisfy the favored criteria, but insist that once we have spelled out what else would then need to be true of her, it is no longer clear that her obedient actions aren't autonomous.
(iii) Accept the claim that Fatma's obedient actions aren't autonomous, but insist that they could still be motivated by an autonomously formed desire. The idea here would be that Fatma might have an autonomous desire to act nonautonomously.[12]

Kristinsson argues that of the four prominent content-neutral accounts of autonomy that he considers (those developed by Christman, Elster, Dworkin, and Frankfurt) none can exploit any of these strategies.[13] Leaving aside his discussion of Frankfurt (on the grounds that Frankfurt's account is, as was argued in Chapter 3, properly understood as an account of identification rather than of autonomy), it transpires that Kristinsson's criticisms of the other three content-neutral accounts of autonomy are only half-persuasive.

Kristinsson notes that for Christman a person is autonomous with respect to a desire "just in case the person who has it would not be motivated to resist it if she were to reflect, with 'minimal internalist rationality'. . .and without self-deception, on the process by which it developed."[14] Kristinsson correctly notes that Christman cannot exploit option (i) to show that on his account Fatma is not autonomous with respect to her desires to obey, since given her values it is perfectly possible that were she to be reflecting in accordance with the conditions that Christman outlines she would not resist its development. Option (ii) is also precluded for Christman, because even if he claimed that for a person to be autonomous with respect to her actions they must be in harmony with her outlook (i.e., if this supplement was added to Christman's account), Fatma would still clearly lack autonomy with respect to her actions. Finally, Kristinsson claims that option (iii) is closed to Christman also, "if only because Christman's theory contains no separate account of autonomous action."[15]

Kristinsson gives similarly short shrift to the content-neutral accounts of autonomy offered by Elster and Dworkin. According to Elster, a person will be heteronomous with respect to any preference that is formed adaptively, that is, that is formed under conditions whereby "a restriction of feasible options leads the person to come to prefer those to the unfeasible ones."[16] Since what matters on Elster's account is not the object of the desires that have been adaptively formed but the way in which they came about his account is a content-neutral one. However, argues Kristinsson, even though Elster might pursue option (i) and claim that Fatma's desires have been formed adaptively and so she is not autonomous with respect to them, it is possible to imagine that her preferences were not adaptive. She might, for example, have simply been "created like this, an adult fully equipped with submissive preferences."[17] Elster also cannot exploit option (ii), for even if Fatma's preferences were nonadaptive this would give us no reason to suppose that she was autonomous with respect to them. Finally, argues Kristinsson, if Elster were to admit that Fatma was not autonomous with respect to her obedient actions, he could still insist that, if formed nonadaptively, she is autonomous with respect to her desire to obey—although this would require that he offer a *substantive* account of what it is for a person to be autonomous with respect to her actions.[18]

Having criticized the views of Christman and Elster, Kristinsson turns to those of Dworkin. For Dworkin, a person is autonomous if she is able to reflect critically upon her first-order desires or preferences, and to change them after such reflection if she so desires. Such reflection must be procedurally independent, free from influences that would subvert the critical reflection of the person concerned.[19] It is clear that Dworkin cannot exploit option (i) to account for Fatma's heteronomy. Nor can he exploit option (ii), for even if Fatma reflectively endorses her submissive attitudes her actions are still under the control of others and not herself. And nor, claims Kristinsson, can Dworkin exploit option (iii), for Dworkin takes autonomy to be a global property of a person's life, or a span thereof, rather than a property of person's desires or actions.[20] Moreover, claims Kristinsson, Dworkin's account of autonomy "provides no grounds for claiming that unconditionally obedient actions necessarily lack autonomy. . . Fatma could obey unconditionally while exercising her ability to reflect with procedural independence on the motivating desire."[21]

Kristinsson is right that Christman, Elster, and Dworkin cannot exploit options (i) or (ii) to account for Fatma's lack of autonomy with respect to her actions. But they can exploit option (iii). Although Kristinsson correctly notes that Christman's account of autonomy does not include an account of what it is for a person to be autonomous with respect to her actions that is separate from his account of what it is for a person to be autonomous with respect to her desires, this does not show that such an account is not available to him. As such, Christman could exploit option (iii) simply by claiming that a person's being autonomous with respect to her desires is necessary but not sufficient for her to be autonomous with respect to her actions. He could thus hold that while Fatma is autonomous with respect to her desires, she is heteronomous with respect to her actions—perhaps because they (and unlike, arguably, her desires) are under the control of others. Kristinsson admits that a similar response could be offered by a defender of Elster's account. However, he claims that Dworkin is precluded from also offering this response since he considers autonomy to be a property of persons with respect to their lives over "a significant period of time," rather than of persons with respect to their "individual actions or desires."[22] This is certainly true of Dworkin's view of autonomy as he outlines it in *The Theory and Practice of Autonomy*, which Kristinsson cites. But it is not true of his earlier account of autonomy in which he was concerned with providing an account of when a person is autonomous with respect to her motivations, her "decisions, motives, desires, habits, and so forth."[23] Since this is so, Dworkin's account of autonomy could be rescued from Kristinsson's criticisms in the same way that Christman's could be, by holding that meeting the procedural conditions that Dworkin outlines is necessary but not sufficient for a person to be autonomous with respect to her actions.[24] Thus, a person who defends Dworkin's account of autonomy along these lines could claim, whereas Fatma is autonomous with respect to her desires to be obedient she is not autonomous with respect to her consequent actions.[25]

Yet although these defenses of Christman's, Elster's and Dworkin's models of autonomy quell Kristinsson's criticisms of them they do so in a way that provides only cold comfort to a defender of the view that the correct analysis of autonomy will be a content-neutral one. They thus do not undermine Kristinsson's aim of moving "Toward a Weakly Substantive Account of Autonomy."[26] It was argued previously that, like Elster, both Christman and Dworkin could add to their accounts of what it is for a person to be autonomous with respect to her first-order desires a separate account of what it is for a person to be autonomous with respect to her actions, where the former might be necessary but not sufficient for the latter. If so, it was argued, these accounts could, like Elster's, avoid Kristinsson's criticisms, for their proponents would not then be committed to claiming that Fatma was autonomous with respect to her actions. However, to offer this argument in defense of these models of autonomy is to concede to Kristinsson that a purely content-neutral analysis of autonomy would be unable to account for the view that Fatma is paradigmatically heteronomous with respect to her actions. This is because for the additional account of what it is for a person to be autonomous with respect to her actions to account for Fatma's heteronomy it must be one that requires that, to be autonomous with respect to her actions, a person must not cede control over them to another agent. Thus, to respond to Kristinsson's criticisms the defenders of the analyses of autonomy offered by Chrisman, Elster, and Dworkin must supplement them with a *substantive* account of what it is for a person to be autonomous with respect to her actions, whereby a person is precluded from being autonomous with respect to her actions if the effective first-order desire that moves her to perform them is one with the content "do whatever the person I am ceding control over my actions to requires me to do."[27] Hence, to avoid Kristinsson's criticisms the defenders of these analyses of autonomy should cease insisting that "there are no a priori constraints on the content of the desires or values that might motivate an autonomous action," and, instead, accept that they are committed to the view that there is at least one.[28]

However, the necessity of conceding that these models of autonomy cannot be content-neutral models if they are to avoid committing their proponents to the unacceptable claim that persons such as Fatma are paradigms of autonomy is not as striking as it might at first appear. This is so for two reasons. First, as was noted previously, to avoid counterexamples such as that of Fatma the proponents of these models of autonomy must hold that persons cannot be autonomous with respect to actions that they are motivated to perform by desires with certain objects, namely, that of ceding control over the actions in question to another. They thus must accept that there is at least one a priori constraint "on the content of the desires or values that might motivate an autonomous action." Second, and more generally, it should be noted that on both Christman's and Dworkin's accounts of autonomy it is necessary for a person to be autonomous with respect to her "decisions, motives, desires, habits, and so forth" that she either counterfactually (Christman), or actually (Dworkin), reflects upon them and either fails to repudiate them (Christman) or endorses them (Dworkin).[29] It is thus necessary on both these accounts that, to be autonomous, a person must value engaging in some degree of critical reflection.[30] As such, then both Christman's and Dworkin's analyses of autonomy are substantive, and not content-neutral, analyses. And these two points can be generalized. Thus, any plausible analysis of autonomy must incorporate two substantive requirements. First, it must require that at least one a priori restriction be placed upon "the content of the desires or values that might motivate an autonomous action": that persons cannot be autonomous with respect to actions that they are motivated to perform by desires with the object of ceding control over the actions in question to another. Second, given the discussion in Chapter 1 of the necessity of using a person's engagement in critical reflection to distinguish her agential desires and actions from those that she was autonomous with respect to, it must require that autonomous persons critically reflect upon their desires and values to some degree, and hence value such reflection. (Both of these requirements are met by the account of practical autonomy developed in Chapter 1.) It should be noted, however, that these substantive requirements are *minimally* substantive requirements, requiring only that autonomous persons retain control over their own actions and engage in some degree of critical reflection. As such, they are compatible with persons being autonomous with respect to a wide range of values. (Indeed, on this account a person could even be autonomous with respect to his abandonment of autonomy.) They thus pose no bar to the minimally substantive account of practical autonomy developed in Chapter 1 playing the central role in bioethical discussions in a contemporary pluralist society.

## IS MORE SUBSTANCE REQUIRED?

Despite appearances, then, the account of practical autonomy that was developed in Chapter 1 is a minimally substantive one. Yet the minimal substance of this account of autonomy could still be considered a theoretical weakness by persons who believe that analyses of autonomy should be more evaluatively laden than this. First, it could be held that the substance of this account of autonomy is too thin, and, as such, it still fails adequately to capture the implicit normative presuppositions that undergird the concept of autonomy. That is, it could be held that this model of practical autonomy should be rejected because only robustly substantive models of autonomy are plausible. Second, it still seems subject to the criticism that it fails to recognize that it is partially constitutive of the concept of autonomy that an autonomous person must be capable of detecting and appropriately responding to certain values or reasons.[31] That is, it could be held that this model of practical autonomy should be rejected because only normative competence models of autonomy are plausible.

## Richardson's Arguments for Robustly Substantive Autonomy

The first set of arguments for a robustly substantive approach to autonomy that will be considered here are those that have been developed by Henry Richardson. Richardson argues that no contemporary analysis of autonomy is a content-neutral analysis, for they are all based upon tacit normative presuppositions.[32] Richardson's argumentative strategy for this conclusion is both elegant and, at first sight, effective. He begins by describing pairs of examples of persons. For each pair of examples one of the persons described is a paradigm case of someone who is autonomous, and the other is a paradigm case of someone who is nonautonomous. Richardson constructs each pair of examples in such a way that although both of the persons described possess the same motivational structure they differ in the values that they are pursuing. As both persons in each pair possess the same formal, content-neutral motivational structures Richardson argues that the explanation for why one person in each pair is paradigmatically autonomous and the other is paradigmatically nonautonomous must lie in values that they pursue. Since this is so, he argues, content-neutral analyses of autonomy necessarily underdescribe the conditions that must be met for a person to be autonomous. And this, Richardson claims, shows that any satisfactory analysis of autonomy must be a robustly substantive analysis of autonomy, whose proponents recognize that "there are *a priori* truths about the content of the values pursued in autonomous action."[33]

The first pair of examples that Richardson develops includes the anthropomorthic fox that Jon Elster uses to exemplify his analysis of adaptive desires and the egotistical lawyer Bully Stryver from Charles Dickens's *A Tale of Two Cities*.[34] After seeing some appealing grapes Elster's fox comes to desire them. On realizing that he cannot reach them, to salve his frustration the fox self-deceptively convinces himself that they were sour, and so he did not want them anyway. The fox was not autonomous with respect to his adaptive preference not to eat the grapes because it arose through self-deception, and persons are paradigmatically nonautonomous with respect to preferences that arise in this way. Similarly, Bully Stryver's preferences concerning his marital intentions also resulted from self-deception. When Lucie Manette turned down his proposal of marriage he denies both to himself and to others that he ever wished to marry her, and ceases to woo her. Just like Elster's fox, then, Stryver self-deceptively adapted his preferences to conform better to his situation once he realized that he could not satisfy those that he originally (and non-self-deceptively) possessed. However, Richardson claims that, unlike Elster's fox, "the autonomy of Stryver's choice to turn away from Lucie is not defeated by his self-deception."[35] According to Richardson, persons must shield themselves from some losses, even through self-deception, to preserve their self-respect. This, Richardson argues, is because self-respect is a necessary condition of autonomy, for without it a person would not believe that her values were worthy of pursuit. Stryver, then, according to Richardson, remains autonomous in a way that Elster's fox does not, for Stryver's self-deception was required to protect his autonomy. Thus, Richardson concludes, since both Elster's fox and Bully Stryver came to possess their desires in the same way, the explanation for why Stryver is held to be autonomous with respect to his relevant desire and why the fox is not must lie in the fact that their respective acts of self-deception were of differing value for them.

The second pair of examples that Richardson considers involves the title character of Frank Capra's *Mr. Smith Goes to Washington*, and Dr. Pangloss, the philosopher in Voltaire's *Candide*. Richardson notes that Mr. Smith's adherence to his idealistic point of view and his refusal to yield to the manipulations of the corrupt Washington powerbrokers exemplifies an autonomous man's constancy to a set of guiding ideals. In contrast to this, Dr. Pangloss's refusal to abandon the Leibnizian doctrine that this is the best of all possible worlds exemplifies not autonomy but a person in the grip of an ideology that has taken over his life. Richardson observes that if these intuitive ascriptions of autonomy and heteronomy are correct, "then it is difficult to escape the conclusion that the difference between Mr. Smith, an exemplar of autonomy, and Dr. Pangloss, an exemplar of pigheadedness, depends at least in part upon the relative soundness of their conceptions of the good, upon whether the ideals they are sticking to are reasonable."[36]

Richardson's third pair of examples consists of two stereotypes: the Cowboy and the Ruthless Lothario. The Cowboy is "a straightforward, nonintellectual person of independent mind who goes his own way, disdains the demands of routinized authority structures, and cares little for what people say about him." The Ruthless Lothario is also a nonconformist, "impervious to the pressures of socialization," who "cares not a whit either for social convention limiting sexual practices or for the feelings of the women he seduces."[37] Yet despite their motivational structures being identical, whereas the Cowboy is an exemplar of autonomy the Ruthless Lothario fails to be autonomous, for his desires "are in the unrestrained service of base sexual ends." Instead of admiring his single-mindedness, then, "We are more likely to think of him as a sort of monster wholly in the grip of desire than as a paragon of self-rule."[38] Again, since the Cowboy and the Ruthless Lothario possess the same formal content-neutral motivational structures Richardson argues that the explanation for why the former is paradigmatically autonomous and the latter is not must lie in the fact that they pursue differing values.

Finally, Richardson contrasts the case of Mary Tyler Moore's social conformist television character Mary Richards with Valmont, the libertine in Stendhal's *Les Liaisons Dangereuses*. Richardson quotes Richard Double's quotation of Mary Richards as saying "I know that it's foolish to care about what other people think, but I do care. That's just the kind of person I am."[39] Richardson agrees with Double that Mary Richards could be autonomous with respect to her adoption of this conformist stance, noting that "A neutralist might attempt to capture this kind of case by holding that self-consciously acknowledged conformity is compatible with autonomy."[40] In contrast to this, Richardson offers the example of Valmont's seduction of the innocent Madame de Tourvel under the instruction of the wicked Madame de Merteuil. When Mme. de Merteuil bullies Valmont into breaking off the affair with the woman whom he now loves, he can only repeat "It is beyond my control. It is beyond my control," in response to Mme. De Tourvel's piteous cries of "why?" Like Mary Richards, Valmont acknowledges his conformity and acquiesces to it, rather than merely accepting it. Unlike Mary Richards, however, such acquiescence does not intuitively render Valmont autonomous with respect to his conformity with the desires of Mme. de Merteuil. Since this is so, Richardson claims, our intuitive ascriptions of autonomy and heteronomy respectively to these characters depend upon the value schemes to which they have acquiesced. And, as such, autonomy must be recognized to be a robustly substantive concept.

## Responding to Richardson

Richardson's pairs of examples fail to prove that the concept of autonomy rests on tacit normative presuppositions, which can only be accounted for by endorsing a robustly substantive account of autonomy. In two of Richardson's pairs of examples the persons in them are equally autonomous, or nonautonomous. This undermines Richardson's claim that the difference in the degree of autonomy that is ascribed to them can only be explained by reference to the different values that each is pursuing. In the other two cases, where the persons in the examples do indeed exhibit differing degrees of autonomy, this difference is best explained not by reference to the different values that they are pursuing but by differences in the processes by which they came to possess their desires.

In Richardson's examples of the Elster's fox and Bully Stryver, and Mr. Smith and Dr. Pangloss, each person in each of these pairs is just as autonomous or heteronomous as their partner. In his discussion of Elster's fox and Bully Stryver, Richardson correctly notes that since the change in the fox's desires arose as a result of self-deception the fox is not autonomous with respect to them. However, Richardson is wrong to claim that Stryver's autonomy is not similarly undermined by his equally self-deceptive acquisition of his desire not to marry Lucie Manette. Richardson argues that Stryver's self-deceptive acquisition of the preference to cease courting Lucie does not undermine his autonomy with respect to this preference because in adapting his desires in this way Stryver, unlike Elster's fox, is preserving his self-respect that is a necessary condition for him to be autonomous. Richardson's argument here is thus based upon the claim that for any preference P possessed by an agent A at time t that is instrumentally valuable in that A's possession of P serves to protect his ability to exercise his autonomy at time t + n, A is autonomous with respect to P. However, not only does

Richardson fail to provide any argument as to why this claim is true, there is good reason to believe that it is false.

To see this, consider the case of a person who wishes to be a slave. A benevolent neurosurgeon who values autonomy highly hears of this and inculcates a preference into him not to sign the slavery contract that he would otherwise accept. This preference becomes operative whenever the would-be slave is moved to sign the contract, and, to be effective, it is so much stronger than his desire to sign that it invariably overwhelms it. The person into whom this preference is inculcated, however, still wishes to become a slave and struggles mightily against this inculcated preference but to no avail. In preventing the would-be slave from becoming a slave this inculcated preference serves to protect him in the exercise of his autonomy. However, insofar as this is not a preference that he decides to satisfy, but merely one to whose operation he is an *entirely* passive bystander, the would-be slave is not autonomous with respect to it. As such, then, Richardson's claim that that any preference P that protects an agent A's exercise of his autonomy at time t + n will be one that A is autonomous with respect to is mistaken. Thus, in discussing Elster's fox and Bully Stryver, Richardson confuses the instrumental value of their respective adaptive preferences to them with respect to the future exercise of their autonomy with the question of whether these individuals are autonomous with respect to their preferences. Insofar as the respective preferences of the fox and of Stryver are formed adaptively, then, both individuals will lack autonomy with respect to them—although Stryver's might be instrumentally valuable to him in a way that the fox's is not to him. Since this is so, then, there is no reason to introduce any normative considerations to explain the purported differences in the degree of autonomy enjoyed by the fox and by Stryver.[41]

A similar point can be made concerning Richardson's discussion of Mr. Smith and Dr. Pangloss. Richardson's intuitions as to why Smith is autonomous with respect to his desire to adhere to his ideals but Pangloss is not are rooted in "the thought that Mr. Smith is acting in a way that better realizes or supports his rational agency than Pangloss is."[42] There are two parts to this intuition: that Smith is more autonomous than Pangloss because his actions *realize* his rational agency and that Smith is more autonomous than Pangloss because his actions *support* it. This latter claim is subject to the same criticism as was Richardson's earlier claim concerning Stryver's autonomy with respect to his adaptive preferences: that the question of whether a person's preference to pursue a certain course of action is instrumentally valuable in supporting the future exercise of his autonomous agency is not the same question as that of whether he was autonomous with respect to the preference in question. Thus, even though Smith's preference to pursue a certain course of action might support his future exercise of his autonomy better than Pangloss's, this has no bearing on whether he is more or less autonomous than Pangloss with respect to them. A different point can be made concerning Richardson's intuition that Smith's course of action better *realizes* his autonomy than Pangloss's realizes his. Richardson is here drawing on the intuition that Pangloss is somehow alienated from his desire to adhere to his principle in a way that Smith is not: he is "in the grip of an ideology." This intuition draws its force from the belief that Smith would deviate from his steadfast adherence to principle were he to be given a good reason to do so (and there just happens not to be any such reasons available), whereas Pangloss could not so deviate because he was so enmeshed in the grip of an ideology that he could not recognize legitimate reasons to abandon it.[43] Yet, as the example is described there is no reason why one *should* hold this belief—although why one might *actually* do so is easily explained. Those who share Richardson's intuitions here are more likely to recognize the appeal of Smith's ideals than those of Pangloss's. Furthermore, persons with this view of the relative merits of these characters' ideals would naturally believe that while Smith had good reason to stick to his position, Pangloss did not. Since this is so, persons who share Richardson's intuitions here are likely to accept his implicit claim that Pangloss's unwillingness to abandon his view was owed to his inability to recognize and act on good reasons in this matter. But it could well be the case that both Smith and Pangloss have equally good reasons for adhering to their positions, with neither having encountered satisfactory arguments to the contrary—and if this is possible then the intuitive force behind Richardson's claim that Smith is autonomous and Pangloss is not dissipates. There is thus no reason to believe that these persons are not both fully autonomous with respect to their respective steadfast adherence to principle, and so there is no difference in autonomy between them to be explained by reference to any tacit normative presuppositions.

Let us now turn to Richardson's pairs of cases in which the persons in each pair do enjoy differing degrees of autonomy. The first pair of cases to be considered here is that of Mary Richards and Valmont. Richardson claims that whereas Mary Richards is intuitively autonomous with respect to her conforming actions, Valmont suffers from diminished autonomy with respect to those actions that he performs at the behest of Mme. de Merteuil. Richardson is correct here. However, the explanation for the difference in the degrees of autonomy exhibited by these persons does not lie in any differing evaluations that might be accorded to the value schemes that they have acquiesced to. Instead, it lies in the ways in which they come to perform their actions. It is clear both from his utterances and from his behavior in the novel that Valmont is under the control of Mme. de Merteuil to the extent that it is she, and not he, who decides which actions he should perform. In this way Valmont is, with respect to his autonomy, in a similar position to Othello as discussed in Chapter 1, for, like Othello, his autonomy with respect to his actions is diminished insofar as another agent is deciding which actions he should perform. Mary Richards, however, is not under the control of another agent in this way. To be sure, she cares about what other people think, and so their views influence her decisions as to which actions she should perform. Yet it is still she, and not someone else, who decides what actions she performs, and so she could still be fully autonomous with respect to her actions in a way that Valmont and Othello could not be. The different degrees of autonomy that are intuitively ascribed to Mary Richards and to Valmont with respect to their actions, then, can readily be explained without recourse to any underlying normative presuppositions about the respective merits of the value schemes to which they acquiesce.

A similar response can be made to Richardson's final pair of examples: the Cowboy and the Ruthless Lothario. Richardson claimed that the Cowboy was autonomous with respect to his desire to "preserve the 'freedom of the range'" because he independently pursued this ideal, regardless of what others might say about him. However, despite being equally cavalier about the opinions of others, the Ruthless Lothario intuitively fails to be autonomous with respect to his desire continually to pursue sexual conquest. This is because, Richardson argued, the value that the Ruthless Lothario was pursuing was not as recognizable as a moral ideal. Yet although Richardson is correct to note that these two individuals intuitively differ with respect to the degree that they are autonomous this difference is rooted not in the differing values that they are pursuing but in the differing processes by which they come to have these values. To see this, it should be noted that while Richardson described the Cowboy as being "of independent mind" the Ruthless Lothario was described as being "simpleminded".[44] This difference is important. If the Cowboy were to be described as simplemindedly following his desire to preserve the freedom of the range and the Ruthless Lothario described as being of independent mind in the pursuit of sexual conquests it seems that Richardson's intuitive ascriptions of autonomy and nonautonomy to these persons would be reversed. Indeed, Richardson implicitly concedes this in a footnote to his discussion where he acknowledges that the apparent nonautonomy of the Ruthless Lothario would not be shared by "a sophisticated and calculating seducer such as Johannes, the character described in Soren Kierkegaard's 'Diary of a Seducer,'" for "the simplemindedness of the Ruthless Lothario is important" for his example to achieve the end that he has designed it for.[45] It is thus clear that what is motivating the intuitive ascriptions of autonomy and nonautonomy to these persons that Richardson draws upon is not the view that "the independent person [must] be pursuing something recognizable as a moral ideal," for Richardson accepts that were the Ruthless Lothario to be "sophisticated and calculating" in the pursuit of sexual conquest he would be autonomous with respect to this.[46] Instead, what is motivating the intuitive ascriptions of autonomy and nonautonomy to the Cowboy and the Ruthless Lothario that Richardson draws upon is the intuition (noted in Chapter 1 and previously) that for a person to be autonomous with respect to her desires she must have engaged in some form of endorsement with respect to them, either of the desires themselves or of the decision-making process that led her to have them. Thus, since the Cowboy is described as being "of independent mind" it intuitively appears that he has endorsed his desires in such a way, and so is autonomous with respect to them, whereas the "simpleminded" (i.e., unreflective) Ruthless Lothario has not, and so is not autonomous with respect to them. But, if this is so, then it is not, as Richardson claims, the difference in the values pursued by the Cowboy and the Ruthless Lothario that explain why the former is autonomous with respect to his desires and the latter is not. Instead, the respective autonomy and heteronomy of these persons can be best explained by reference to the differences in the processes by which they come to be moved by their desires.

## Stoljar's Feminist Intuition

Richardson, then, has failed to show that a satisfactory account of autonomy must be a robustly substantive one, for he has failed to show that ascriptions of autonomy rest on any implicit normative presuppositions about the values that autonomous agents can pursue. A similar argument for the view that any satisfactory account of personal autonomy must be robustly substantive has been offered by Natalie Stoljar. Stoljar argues that content-neutral (and, by extension, minimally substantive) analyses of autonomy are inadequate for they could count as autonomous women whose desires and actions are the products of their internalization of oppressive norms of femininity and whose content and objects thus preclude their possessors from being autonomous with respect to them. Terming the rejection of content-neutral analyses of autonomy for this reason "the feminist intuition," Stoljar supports her view by discussing Kristin Luker's bioethics-related research into the decision-making procedures of a set of women who had internalized misguided norms concerning women's sexuality and whose decisions to take contraceptive risks led to their becoming pregnant and then electing to procure abortions.[47] Stoljar claims that owing to the content of the norms that these women had internalized they could not be autonomous with respect to their decisions to run contraceptive risks, even if they satisfy all of the conditions for autonomy that are required by standard content-neutral analyses of autonomy.[48] From this, Stoljar concludes that "To vindicate the feminist intuition that the subjects [of Lukers's study] are not autonomous, therefore, feminists need to develop a strong substantive theory of autonomy."[49]

Stoljar's argument is unpersuasive. An initial objection to it has been pressed independently by Paul Benson and Diana Meyers, who note that "Critical examination of and resistance to oppression often arise from within," and that "multiply oppressed individuals are in some respects better positioned. . . to exercise autonomous moral and political agency. . .than multiply privileged individuals are."[50] In support of this Meyers holds that robustly substantive theories of autonomy such as those preferred by Stoljar would "deny existing opportunities for choice and. . .erase the real, some-times courageous choices women have actually made."[51] The view here is that, contra Stoljar, that a person has been brought up to accept oppressive social norms does not preclude her from autonomously challenging them. Indeed, such autonomous challenges might, for some individuals, even be stimulated by their recognition that the norms that they are subject to bind them in ways that they do not accept. Despite the initial plausibility of this objection, however, it is indirectly self-defeating. To challenge Stoljar's femi-nist intuition one must offer an example of a person who has *internalized* the norms that she (Stoljar) regards as being inimical to the autonomy of those who possess them and yet who is still autonomous. The objections offered here by Benson and Meyers, however, are based upon examples of persons who are *challenging* the authority of the norms that they have been raised to accept. Such persons will thus not have internalized these norms in the way that Stoljar believes would undermine their autonomy, and so their obvious autonomy cannot serve as the basis for an objection to her view.

Benson is on considerably firmer ground when he observes that not all feminists are likely to endorse Stoljar's "feminist" intuition. Benson notes that the type of social conventions that Stoljar is concerned with do not in themselves prevent women from critically reflecting upon their motivations and modifying them on the basis of such reflection. Moreover, "the effects of their social training have not, *ex hypothesi*, diminished these women's [i.e., those who take ownership of their decisions] regard for their own compe-tence and worth as persons appropriately positioned to present their reasons for acting and to speak with authority in support of their decisions, should others question them."[52] Benson notes that although such women would not offer reasons for taking contraceptive risks that most feminists would accept, this "does not diminish their ability to authorize their decisions and fully inhabit what they do in the sense that autonomy requires."[53] Benson's response to Stoljar here can be buttressed by noting that a woman who has internalized the norms that Stoljar considers to be antithetical to feminism and who makes decisions on the basis of them could still be fully autonomous with respect to her decisions and her actions. To draw both from the discus-sion of the Degree Condition in Chapter 1, and to presage the arguments of Chapter 7, for a person's decisions to be normative for her she must have some reason for making them. Since this is so, the value-set on which she bases her decisions cannot be one that she has simply chosen for herself *de novo*, for, if it were, she would have had no reason to prefer this value-set over any other, and so she would not have any reason to prefer the deci-sions that she makes on its basis to any other decisions that she could have made. To be autonomous, then—that is, for her decisions to be normative for her—a person must possess a value-set that is (at least partially) outside her control. But this is a requirement that could be met by (almost) any value-set, whether feminist or not.[54] Thus, even if a woman is socialized into a non-feminist value-set, provided that she meets the Threshold Condition and the Degree Condition (outlined in Chapter 1) with respect to her making of her decisions there seems to be no intuitive rationale for holding her to be heteronomous with respect to her decisions and the actions that they directly lead her to perform. Absent further argument from Stoljar, then, there is no reason not to consider the women in Lukers's study to be autonomous with respect to their decisions to take contraceptive risks. Stoljar thus cannot support her claim that a robustly substantive account of autonomy is needed to accommodate her feminist intuition, especially since it is far from clear that this intuition would be shared by all feminists.

As well as offering reasons why Stoljar's argument in favor of a robustly substantive account of autonomy should not be accepted, Benson also offers reasons as to why such an approach to analyzing autonomy should be rejected. Echoing Dworkin, Benson notes that to hold that to be autonomous persons must accept certain values would lead to "far-reaching skepticism about our ordinary prospects for autonomy"—a price associated with accepting robustly substantive accounts of autonomy that Benson considers to be too costly.[55] More substantively, Benson argues that the proponents of robustly substantive accounts of autonomy conflate "the power to *take ownership* of one's actions with something quite different, the power to *get things right*, or the ability to adopt the preferences or values one ought to have (or at least avoid those one ought not to have)."[56] That is, holds Benson, the proponents of such accounts confuse the ideal of orthonomy, *right* rule, with the ideal of autonomy, *self*-rule. That these are different ideals can be seen, argues Benson, from the fact that "we can autonomously take ownership of our mistakes and limitations and act autonomously when bounded by them, even when we are not entirely capable of doing precisely the right thing for just the right reasons."[57]

A final reason for rejecting Stoljar's robustly substantive approach to autonomy can be drawn from Marina A. L. Oshana's example of the Would-Be Surrendered Woman, which she uses for another purpose.[58] What this woman wants most is to "surrender to the strong direction, or at least the strong arms, of a loving man," but, owing to her circumstances, she is instead "a self-supporting, successful professional woman," who has simply become "autonomous by accident."[59] Despite having internalized norms that Stoljar would no doubt consider to be inimical to her autonomy, the Would-Be Surrendered Woman is fully autonomous, even if she does not wish to be. As such, it seems that it cannot be the case that the content of the norms that a person has internalized is sufficient to render her nonautonomous with respect to those of her decisions that flow from them. In response to this a defender of a robustly substantive approach to analyzing autonomy might charge that the example of the Would-Be Surrendered Woman is inappropriate, in that it is her fate to be so situated that she is unable to make decisions on the basis of her misguided norms of femininity—and were she able to do so she would lose the autonomy that she currently possesses. Yet to respond in this way will not only run afoul of Benson's second objection, given previously, it will also run afoul of an objection that has been offered by John Santiago. Santiago argues that Stoljar's feminist intuition seems to point not to difficulties with the contents of the norms that the women in Lukers's study have internalized but "with features of the social system in which these agents reside and their position within it."[60] After all, he notes, "many *men* adhere to and act upon . . . [these norms] . . . they raise their daughters to become mothers, act more respectfully to married women with children than those without, and so on. Yet it is unlikely that the feminist intuition would be appropriate in such cases, for we hardly think they are less autonomous in virtue of holding [such norms]. . ."[61] Stoljar's feminist intuition, then, cannot serve as the foundation for a robustly substantive approach to analyzing personal autonomy.

## NORMATIVE COMPETENCE THEORIES OF AUTONOMY

If there is reason not to accept the robustly substantive approach to analyzing personal autonomy that is favored by Richardson and Stoljar, what then of the plausibility of normative competence theories of autonomy, which, like their robustly substantive cousins, have also been developed as alternatives to the type of minimally substantive accounts of autonomy such as that developed in Chapter 1?

Normative competence theories of autonomy are more minimally substantive than robustly substantive accounts of autonomy for they "need not entail any direct, normative restrictions on the contents of autonomous agents' preferences or values."[62] Indeed, they "allow that normatively competent persons can choose what is unreasonable or wrong or value what is bad, because competence lies some distance short of perfect evaluative perception or responsiveness."[63] As such, then, they do not run afoul of the objections to robustly substantive theories of autonomy of the sort developed by Richardson and Stoljar. Despite this, however, they should still be rejected. To see why, consider Thomas Hill Jr.'s endorsement of Rousseau's view that a person cannot coherently consent to being enslaved, since "a person's consent releases others from obligation only if it is autonomously given, and consent resulting from underestimation of one's moral status is not autonomously given."[64] For Hill, then, to be autonomous a person must be able to detect and respond appropriately to the value that he has as a human being, where to respond appropriately to such a value is to repudiate one's own enslavement. But it is not clear why the repudiation of being enslaved must be the appropriate response to the recognition of one's moral status. Indeed, a coherent case could be made that it would be rational for a person with certain desires and values to endorse his own enslavement, even if he did not underestimate his own moral status.[65] More pointedly, consider Satan's embrace of his fate with the words "Evil, be thou my good."[66] Even though Satan's response to evil is inappropriate (and conceptually so) he is not therefore rendered nonautonomous with respect to his desires and actions. In fact, Milton's Satan seems to be a paradigm of an autonomous, self-directed individual. From these two examples it is clear that the claim that to be autonomous a person must respond "appropriately" to the reasons or values that she detects is too strong, for neither the reflective slave nor Milton's Satan obviously fail to be autonomous with respect to their slavish or pro-evil desires.[67]

In response to this, a proponent of the normative competence approach to autonomy could retreat to the claim that to be autonomous a person must be able to *detect* certain reasons and values, leaving it open how she could respond to them. But this weaker response will not serve as an adequate ground for a theory of autonomy. First, it is incomplete, for its proponents will need to provide an account of which reasons and values must be detected by a person for her to be autonomous. Second, it is not clear why one would accept that the mere ability to detect certain reasons and values would be necessary for a person to be autonomous. On this modified normative competence approach to autonomy, it would be necessary for a person to be autonomous that she detect certain reasons and values even if such reasons and values would never have any bearing upon her motivations or her actions. As such, it is unclear why her ability to detect the reasons or values in question would be relevant to the question of whether she was autonomous with respect to her motivations and actions.

This second general objection to the normative competence approach to analyzing autonomy leads to the third: that it is not clear why persons should be required to detect any particular values at all. It is, for example, possible to imagine a person who systematically fails to detect the reasons or values that the proponent of a normative competence model of autonomy requires him to detect, and yet whose decisions flow from his own preference structure, and arise from a procedure that he has reflected upon and is satisfied with, and which directly motivate his actions, free from the interference of others. It would thus appear that there is no reason to hold that such a self-directing person fails to be autonomous with respect to his desires and actions. The normative competence approach to analyzing autonomy, then, should be rejected.

## CONCLUSION

The previous arguments have served to clarify the relationship between autonomy and normativity. From the discussion of Kristinsson's objections to content-neutral accounts of autonomy it is clear that no such account of autonomy will be theoretically satisfactory. Given both this and the discussion in Chapter 1 of the necessity for autonomy of critical reflection it is clear that the account of practical autonomy that was developed in that earlier chapter is not, despite first appearances, a content-neutral account, but a minimally substantive one. Yet that this account of autonomy is a minimally substantive one does not preclude it from being able to play the central role accorded to autonomy in contemporary bioethics. Its minimal substantive commitments do not preclude it from recognizing as autonomous persons with diverse value commitments, and so it would still be an appropriate value to draw on in developing a framework for discussions of bioethical and medical issues within a pluralistic society. With this point in hand, then, it is now time to turn in the remainder of this part of this volume to consider the relationship that this account of practical autonomy has with two other concepts with which it is often coupled in discussions of bioethics: choice and constraint.

# 6 Autonomy and Choice

## INTRODUCTION

It is generally believed that, from the point of view of persons who hold autonomy to be valuable, a person's having more choices is better than her having fewer.[1] It has, for example, been argued by some bioethicists that persons who value autonomy should be in favor of markets in human kidneys and ova,[2] commercial surrogate pregnancy,[3] elective amputation and radical cosmetic surgery,[4] and prenatal genetic diagnosis.[5] The view that persons who value autonomy should prefer persons to have more choices rather than fewer has, however, recently been subject to a great deal of criticism.[6] Indeed, rather than holding that persons who value autonomy should favor persons having more choices rather than fewer, it is now widely believed that they should favor the *absence* of certain types of choices from persons' choice-sets—that is, that they should favor persons having *fewer* choices rather than more. Three types of arguments are mustered in support of this initially counterintuitive conclusion: arguments from constraining options, arguments from irresistible offers, and arguments from ambivalence-inducing temptation. In this chapter each of these arguments will be considered in turn, and, in so doing, it will be shown that none of them successfully establish that a valuer of autonomy should favor persons having fewer options rather than more. The argument in this chapter is not, however, a purely negative one. In responding to these three types of arguments in favor of the view that a valuer of autonomy should favor persons having fewer choices rather than more the relationship between autonomy and choice will become clear. Indeed, it will be argued that in certain *very specific cases* a valuer of autonomy should indeed prefer persons to have fewer options rather than more—although for reasons that are different in kind from those offered by the proponents of the standard arguments in favor of this conclusion.[7]

Before progressing to the arguments, however, three caveats are in order. First, the claim that is being addressed in this chapter is that persons who value *autonomy* should favor persons having fewer choices rather than more, and not the distinct claim that those who are concerned with human *well-being* should favor persons having fewer choices rather than more.[8] Second, in the following discussion of constraining options, irresistible offers, and tempting offers, the types of options and offers that are at issue will be illustrated by reference to discussions in which their presence within persons' choice-sets is used by the authors who draw on them to support particular normative conclusions. The use of such references to illustrate the types of options that are at issue should not, however, be understood to imply that the normative conclusions that their authors intend to support are correct.[9] The aim of this chapter is not to argue for any particular normative conclusions concerning issues such as kidney sales or whether there should be restrictions imposed on the availability of antibiotics but to establish the relationships that hold between practical autonomy and the availability of choices. Third, although the participants in the discussions of autonomy and choice in both autonomy theory and bioethics often take themselves simply to be focusing on the effects that certain choices have on a person's autonomy, this gloss obscures an important distinction between the effects that choices might have on a person's autonomy simpliciter, and the effects that they might have on her ability to *use* her autonomy effectively. If a choice adversely affects a person's autonomy simpliciter it will render her less autonomous with respect to (some or all) of her actions subsequent either to its mere appearance in her choice-set, or subsequent to her choice of it.[10] For example, the choice to take a high dose of the "zombie drug" scopolamine would be a choice whose pursuit would be likely to render the chooser less autonomous with respect to some of her subsequent actions. If a choice adversely affects a person's ability to use her autonomy effectively it will not render less autonomous in any way but will render her less able to use her autonomy to achieve her goals or satisfy her desires. For example, a person whose elective plastic surgery goes awry will not thereby be rendered less autonomous with respect to her subsequent actions but will be unable to use her autonomy to pursue a successful career as a model.[11] Similarly, a person who is faced with a range of alternatives that he finds unpalatable (such as, for example, the option to sell a kidney or remain in poverty) will not be able to use his autonomy as effectively as would a person whose option-set was palatable to him, but this does not show that the former person is any less autonomous simpliciter than the latter.[12] Distinguishing between the effects that choices might have on a person's autonomy *simpliciter*, and the effects that they might have on her ability to *use* her autonomy effectively is important, both for the sake of conceptual clarity and also because these different ways in which choices might adversely affect a person's autonomy will not both be of concern to valuers of autonomy. If a person values autonomy intrinsically (and not instrumentally) then she will be concerned only with the effect that a person's choices would have on her autonomy simpliciter. If, however, a person values autonomy instrumentally (and not intrinsically), then she would be concerned both with the effects that a person's choices would have on her autonomy simpliciter, and with the effects that they would have on her ability to use her autonomy effectively—*provided that* the person in question was not autonomously choosing to trade off her autonomy to secure some good that she valued more. (A person who valued autonomy instrumentally would not, for example, be concerned with a person's decision to enter a monastic order and submit his will to that of an abbot in order to secure the life of religious devotion that he considered to be his vocation, for she would accept that such a person could be trading off her autonomy for a good that she valued more.) Although these theoretical differences (between a person's choices having an effect of her autonomy simpliciter, and having an effect on her ability to use it, and between the intrinsic and instrumental evaluation of autonomy) are often overlooked in discussions of autonomy and choice, care will be taken in the following discussion to make it clear both how a choice is supposed adversely to affect a person's autonomy (i.e., simpliciter, or with respect to her ability to use it), and hence which type of valuer of autonomy would be concerned with it.

## CONSTRAINING OPTIONS

One of the standard arguments in favor of the view that, from the point of view of a person who values autonomy, a person's having more choices can be worse than her having fewer, is the argument from constraining options. According to the proponents of such an argument the presence of certain options within persons' choice-sets is likely to lead to their autonomy being compromised, rather than their ability to exercise it being enhanced. This is because the choice of certain options would lead to persons being less able to exercise their autonomy than they would have been able to had that option not been chosen. (As such, this argument is aimed at persons who value autonomy instrumentally.) Such arguments are of three main types: those that focus upon options that, if chosen, are likely to impair the ability of *the person who chooses them* to exercise her own autonomy post-choice; those that focus upon options that, if chosen, are likely to impair the ability of persons *other* than the persons who chose them to exercise their autonomy; and, finally, those that, if chosen, are likely to impair the ability of *both* the person who choose them, *and* other persons who do not, to exercise their autonomy.

### Individual Constraining Options

A version of the first of these arguments for the conclusion that, from the point of view of a person who instrumentally values autonomy persons would be better off having fewer choices rather than more has been developed by Paul M. Hughes in support of the conclusion that persons should not have the option to sell a nonvital organ, such as a kidney.[13] For Hughes, such an option would be an individual constraining option because it is likely that a person who chose it would consequently suffer from a constrained choice-set post-sale, and so would be less able effectively to exercise her autonomy to satisfy her own desires or pursue her own goals that she was prior to the sale of her organ. This is because, claims Hughes, such a sale is likely to be physically debilitating to the vendor, and thus would make it even harder for him to secure the sort of employment that is available to him. As such, the sale of an organ is likely to reinforce the vendor's impoverishment, especially if it was sold to pay off debts, or to supply a dowry, in that it would make is less likely that he would be able to escape his autonomy-limiting economic circumstances.[14] Thus, since the sale of a nonvital organ would typically not enrich a vendor in a way that would increase the number of options available to him, but would, instead, be likely to lead to their diminution owing to his physical debilitation, the sale of a (e.g.) kidney, argues Hughes, would serve to diminish, rather than enhance, a person's ability to use his autonomy effectively post-sale. As such, then, concludes Hughes, the option to sell a nonvital organ is an individual constraining option, and so persons who value autonomy should oppose its presence within persons' choice-sets.[15]

Before moving to consider how group constraining options are supposed to work to compromise the autonomy of those persons in whose option-sets they are present, it is important to note that Hughes's argument must be addressed to persons who value autonomy instrumentally, for it is not the case that a person will be rendered less autonomous with respect to some or all of her actions as a result of selling a nonvital organ; it will still be she, and not someone else, who is directing her actions post-sale, even if Hughes is correct to claim that the range of options that she has available to her post-sale will be narrowed. Hughes's argument thus rests on the (plausible) assumption that a person who sells a nonvital organ is not in doing so deliberately trading off a degree of her autonomy through to secure some other good that she prefers but wishes only to trade off an organ for another good (e.g., money).

## Group Constraining Options

With the outline of Hughes's argument against organ sales in hand it is clear why he believes that, from the point of view of a person who values autonomy, having more choices is not always better than having fewer. It is also clear why the proponents of another type of argument from constraining options, the argument from group constraining options, believe this, too. As was discussed previously, an individual constraining option is an option that, if chosen, is likely to be autonomy-limiting for the person who chooses it. By contrast, a group constraining option is an option that, if chosen, is likely either not to affect the autonomy of the person who chooses it, or enhance his ability to exercise it—but at the cost of limiting the ability of other persons in the same choice-situation that the chooser was in (i.e., prior to his choosing the option in question) to exercise their autonomy. T. L. Zutlevics argues that giving persons in impoverished countries the option of selling a nonvital organ would be a group constraining option of this sort.[16] Unlike Hughes, Zutlevics accepts that the sale of (e.g.) a kidney might enhance the ability of an impoverished person from a developing country to exercise her autonomy post-sale.[17] Despite this, however, she argues that allowing a trade in organs in which persons from poor countries act as vendors and persons from wealthy countries act as buyers would serve to constrain the ability of other persons who are in the same choice-situation as the vendors. Zutlevics argues that allowing such a trade would encourage wealthy countries to refrain from providing aid to the developing countries from which such vendors would be drawn so that they could ensure that they would continue to provide them with a ready supply of cheap transplantable organs. Since this is so, she claims, while the option of selling a kidney might not be an individual constraining option, it would be a *group* constraining option, for, if chosen, it would result in persons other than the vendors suffering from limitations on their ability to exercise their autonomy in ways that they would not have otherwise suffered from.[18] Thus, she concludes, from the point of view of a valuer of autonomy it would be better were persons not to have such group constraining options available to them.[19]

## Ultimate Constraining Options

In the discussion of constraining options it was the case that *either* the chooser, *or* other persons who are in the same choice-situation that he was in prior to choosing the option in question, would be likely to suffer from limitations on their autonomy as a result of a constraining option being chosen. The final type of constraining option, however, is much more deleterious from the point of view of a valuer of autonomy. Were this type of constraining option to be present in persons' choice-sets it is likely that *both* those who choose it *and* the other members of their relevant group would suffer from limitations on their autonomy. This type of constraining option can thus be dubbed the "ultimate" type of constraining option.

Ultimate constraining options can be illustrated through the possibility of persons having the option to purchase antibiotics at will.[20] It is frequently difficult to determine without laboratory testing whether an ailment is caused by bacterial or viral infection. As such, were antibiotics freely available to persons they would often use them in an attempt to treat diseases whose symptoms were caused by viral rather than bacterial agents. (This is especially so since the most common diseases that people are subject to—colds and influenza—are viral in origin.) Such use of antibiotics is perfectly rational. After all, if the disease in question was bacterial in origin, then treating it with antibiotics is likely to be effective. If, however, it is viral in origin, then the agent who took antibiotics in an attempt to treat it would not be medically worse off for having done so—although they would be slightly worse off financially if they purchased the antibiotics themselves. On the face of it, such self-medication does not seem to be especially problematic. However, things become complicated once it is recognized that "There is a well-known connection between the effectiveness of an antibiotic drug and how commonly it has been used."[21] Were persons to have the option of taking antibiotics at will there would be an increase in the numbers of them that would be taken, and they would frequently be taken in situations where their use was medically inappropriate. This would lead to antibiotics becoming less effective (or even ineffective) with a corresponding increase "in the dangers and costs to which each member of the community would then be exposed because resistant bacteria require stronger, higher-priced drugs to treat, are more likely to require hospitalization, and are much more likely to kill the subjects they infect."[22] Having the option to secure antibiotics unrestrictedly would thus have the effect of an individual constraining option. Although if only one person overused antibiotics to treat her infections she would not thereby by rendered vulnerable to increasing "dangers and costs" through their overuse, since she would be doing so in conjunction with the similar overuse of many other persons, her having the option to take antibiotics unrestrictedly would lead to a situation in which she was subject to increased dangers and costs. Being subject to both more serious illness and additional financial burdens would reduce a person's ability to exercise her autonomy effectively when compared to a situation in which she was not subject to them. As such, the option unrestrictedly to use antibiotics would be an individual constraining option, for it would be likely that a person who had this option within her choice-set would be less able to use her autonomy effectively that would a person who lacked it. Moreover, the option to use antibiotics unrestrictedly would also have the other-regarding effects of a group constraining option, for the autonomy-compromising effect of the presence of this option within a person's choice-set depends not only on her choice to pursue it but on the same choice being made by others. For a person to suffer from a compromised ability to exercise her autonomy effectively as a result of being subject to the increased dangers and costs associated with the overuse of antibiotics it is necessary that not only she but others in her situation decide to overuse them.[23] From the point of view of a valuer of autonomy, then, the option to access antibiotics without restriction should, as an ultimate constraining option, be removed from persons' choice-sets.[24]

## Do Constraining Options Show That Fewer Choices are Better Than More?

At first sight, the arguments from constraining options appear to show that a valuer of autonomy should favor persons having fewer choices rather than more. Yet to draw this conclusion would be too hasty. The three types of constraining options outlined previously are all understood to be autonomy-limiting because, if chosen, *they are likely to limit the number of options that persons would have post-choice for exercising their autonomy.* Thus, an individual constraining option is likely to be an autonomy-limiting option since its choice would be likely to reduce the number of options that would be available to its chooser after its choice. Similarly, a group constraining option is likely to be an autonomy-limiting option since its choice would be likely to reduce the number of options available to members of the chooser's group after its choice, and an ultimate constraining option is autonomy-limiting insofar as its presence within persons' choice-sets is likely to result in both the chooser and the other members of her group having fewer options to choose from. Rather than showing that from the point of view of a valuer of autonomy persons having *fewer* choices can be better than their having more, then, the arguments from constraining options show instead that for a valuer of autonomy having more choices would be better for persons than their having fewer. Thus, insofar as they are offered in support of the claim that from the point of view of a valuer of autonomy it would be better that persons have fewer choices rather than more, such arguments are self-defeating.

## THE ARGUMENTS FROM IRRESISTIBLE OFFERS

The arguments from constraining options thus fail to show that a valuer of autonomy should prefer persons to have fewer choices rather than more, for the force of the arguments is drawn from the (converse) view that a valuer of autonomy should prefer persons having *more* choices rather than fewer. The same is not true, however, of two other types of arguments that are invoked to show that a valuer of autonomy should prefer persons having fewer choices to their having more: the arguments from irresistible offers, and the argument from ambivalence-inducing temptation.

Unlike the arguments from constraining options the arguments from irresistible offers are not based on the view that limiting a person's options at time *t* might serve to ensure that she has a greater number of options at *t+1* than she otherwise would have done. Instead, they are based on the claim that the presence of certain options will *in themselves* serve to compromise the autonomy of those to whom they are made, where such compromise is not a result of any future diminution in the number of options that the persons who choose them would enjoy. Such arguments from irresistible offers can be divided into two main types. The first and simplest of these arguments, the Argument from Literally Irresistible Offers, is based on the claim that, for some persons, certain offers would, quite simply, literally be irresistible. Were such persons not to want to accept the offer, and yet did so anyway as a result of its irresistibility, the presence of this option within their choice-sets would lead to the diminution in their autonomy through leading them to behave nonautonomously.[25] The second argument from irresistibility, the Silencing Argument from Irresistibility, is more subtle. The proponents of this argument first note that certain offers would be far more attractive to persons than any other options in their choice-set. Since this is so, they continue, such favored options would, for the persons faced with them, render ineligible the other options that they would have otherwise pursued through drastically increasing the opportunity costs associated with them. Rather than having several eligible options open to them, then, such persons would only have *one*. The introduction of this option would thus diminish these potential vendors' ability to exercise their autonomy by reducing the number of eligible options that they possess.[26]

## Assessing the Arguments from Irresistible Offers

The Argument from Literally Irresistible Offers is the least persuasive of the arguments from irresistibility, for it is highly unlikely that its first premise would ever be true. It is implausible to claim that some offers would be so literally irresistible that persons could not resist accepting them against their own wills. Certain offers might sing a Siren's song to many, but it is highly unlikely that this song will have the same effect as that of the original Sirens. The Silencing Argument from Irresistibility, however, cannot be so readily dismissed. This argument draws on the intuition that were certain especially attractive offers to occur in persons' choice-sets (e.g., the offer to a desperate graduate student to buy one of her kidneys for two million dollars) then the range of eligible options that they would be faced with would be reduced to one.[27] Since such persons would no longer be able to exercise their autonomy as fully as they could when they could choose from a range of options, a valuer of autonomy should oppose the introduction of such options. Thus, from the point of view of one who values autonomy, fewer options would be better than more.

This argument is certainly plausible. However, like the first, it is fatally flawed. This argument is based on the view that the less eligible options a person has to choose from then the less she will be able to exercise her autonomy. This view of the relationship between a person's ability to exercise her autonomy and her possession of a range of eligible options is plausible owing to the rationalistic overtones of the concept of autonomy, such that a person is exercising his autonomy to a higher degree when he deliberates carefully about the options that are available to him and chooses one on the basis of that deliberation. For persons who accept the rationalistic connotations of the concept of autonomy it makes sense to believe that if a person only has one eligible option available to him (or, more precisely, if he believes that he only has one eligible option available to him) then he will not greatly exercise his autonomy in choosing it.[28] But this view of what is involved in a person exercising his autonomy conflates the *deliberative process* that a person might employ in the exercise of his autonomy with the *exercise* of his autonomy. A person might, for example, simply have no need to deliberate carefully about his potential course of action because the path that he should take is clear to him.[29] This does not imply that such a person acts unthinkingly, as a nonautonomous agent such as a dog or a small child might act. Rather, it simply implies that in this instance he found it easy to discover what course of action he should pursue, and so found it easy to exercise his autonomy effectively. Since this is so, the fact that a person finds one particular course of action to be so appealing that he does not need to deliberate for long prior to choosing it does not show that he thereby suffers from a compromised ability to exercise his autonomy.[30] Thus, the proponents of this argument from irresistibility fail to show that having such an irresistible option in one's choice-set would undermine one's ability to exercise one's autonomy, and hence they fail to show that, from the point of view of a valuer of autonomy, the possibility of such irresistible options shows that more choices can be worse than fewer.

## THE ARGUMENT FROM AMBIVALENCE-INDUCING TEMPTATION

A further argument for the claim that, from the point of view of a valuer of autonomy, a person's having fewer choices is preferable to her having more is based on the claim that persons would be precluded from exercising their autonomy owing to their suffering from a form of motivational ambivalence generated by tempting offers. This type of argument has been offered to oppose legalizing the sale of human transplant kidneys from live vendors and has been discussed in the context of paying human research subjects.[31] The proponents of this argument first note that a person who is suffering from temptation is likely to experience motivational ambivalence. That is, he is likely to be as strongly motivated *not* to perform the act that he is tempted to do, as he is motivated to perform it. Such ambivalence would preclude a person who experiences it from exercising his autonomy, since it would preclude him from having a motivationally unified self to ground his *self*-direction. The proponents of this argument then note that many persons faced with tempting offers would experience such motivational ambivalence. Since this is so, they conclude, respect for autonomy requires that certain offers be eliminated from persons' choice-sets, since they would lead to some persons being precluded from exercising their autonomy as a result of their suffering from such ambivalence.

This Argument from Ambivalence-Inducing Temptation, however, fares no better than the Arguments from Irresistibility. According to the proponents of this argument persons who are ambivalent about pursuing certain options will thereby be precluded from exercising their autonomy. Since this is so, the proponents of this argument conclude, a valuer of autonomy should prefer that such ambivalence-inducing offers do not feature in persons' option-sets, and, hence, should hold that fewer choices can be better than more. As it stands, however, this argument is incomplete, for its conclusion will only follow if autonomy possesses *intrinsic*, and not merely *instrumental*, value. A person who is ambivalent towards an option he is faced with is ambivalent because, given his motivational psychology, both accepting the option and not accepting it are equally attractive to him. Since this is so, when he picks a course of action concerning whether or not to accept he will not be directed in this picking by his motivational- set: his values, desires, pro and con attitudes, and so on. Given that this person is genuinely ambivalent, his motivational-set could just equally have justified the *opposite* course of action to that which he picked. A person in this situation would have no identifiable self to ground his self-direction and so would be precluded from exercising his autonomy. Such preclusion would not matter if the ambivalent person's autonomy were only of *instrumental* value to him, for then his autonomy would be of value to him only in situations when it would matter for him whether it was he, or someone else, who was directing his actions. Were he to be in a situation where it did not matter if it were he or some other person directing his actions, or where it would be preferable from his own point of view for another person to direct his actions, then the exercise of his autonomy would have (respectively) *no* value, or *negative* value, to him. It is the first of these situations that the genuinely ambivalent offeree finds himself in. Since such a person has no reason to choose to accept the offer over choosing to reject it, it does not matter from the point of view of one concerned solely with securing the best outcome for him (i.e., from the point of view of one who is concerned solely with the instrumental value of his autonomy) whether it is he, or someone else, who makes the decision as to whether or not he should accept the offer in question. The instrumental value of the autonomy of a person in such a situation is thus zero. If autonomy were of only instrumental value, then, it would not matter from the point of view of a valuer of autonomy that such an ambivalent person would be precluded from exercising his autonomy when faced with such an offer. Given the motivational-set and epistemic limitations of such a person his autonomy was of no instrumental value to him in this situation anyway.

If one believes that autonomy is only of instrumental value, then, the Argument from Ambivalence-Inducing Temptation has no force. Thus, as was noted previously, for this argument to have force it must rest on the view that autonomy is *intrinsically* valuable. And the more intrinsically valuable one believes autonomy to be the stronger will be this argument from temptation, for the more intrinsically valuable autonomy is the more persons who value it have to decry the existence of options that would undermine it. To complete this argument, then, one must show that autonomy is intrinsically valuable—and to make it a *strong* argument one must show that the intrinsic value of autonomy is high. As will be argued in

Chapter 10, however, there is good reason to believe that autonomy is not intrinsically valuable. (Indeed, this is supported indirectly by the discussion of constraining options, previously, for the force of those arguments rested upon the intuitively plausible assumption that more choice is better then less—and it seems plausible that this is so as it would enable persons to exercise their autonomy so as to fulfill their own desires and achieve their own goals.)[32] At best, then, the Argument from Ambivalence-Inducing Temptation is incomplete—and, at worse, mistaken.

## WHY FEWER CHOICES *COULD* BE BETTER THAN MORE, FOR A VALUER OF AUTONOMY

So far, then, there is no reason to believe that from the point of view of persons who value autonomy persons having fewer choices is preferable to them having more. But, given the arguments offered in response to the Silencing Argument from Irresistibility, given previously, it seems that we also have no reason to accept the view that, from the point of view of a person who values autonomy, *more* options are necessarily *better* than fewer. Indeed, an argument from Gerald Dworkin shows this clearly:

> Suppose someone ranks three goods A, B, and C in that order. Then, making certain plausible assumptions about the infinite divisibility of utility, there will be A, B, and C such that the person prefers a choice between B and C to receiving A. This will occur when the utility of having a choice between B and C plus the utility of B is greater than the utility of A. This seems to me irrational. Leaving aside some special feature about this particular choice, for example, that somebody promised me $1,000 if I made the choice between B and C, why should I prefer to receive my second-ranked alternative to my first?[33]

It is thus clear that, from the point of view of one who values autonomy instrumentally, what matters is the *subjective desirability* of the options that are available to a person rather than the *number* of them. As such, although the standard arguments (outlined previously) that are offered in favor of the view that fewer choices can be preferable to more fail, with respect to a person's ability to exercise her autonomy effectively her having fewer choices *might* be better than her having more.

As Dworkin noted, this will be the case if the choices that are available to her in the former case are those that she would prefer to those in the latter case. It will also be the case if a person prefers to have fewer options rather than more because he knows that he suffers from weakness of will, and would be tempted to pursue options other than those that he believes that he has most reason to pursue were he to be faced with them. Such was the case with certain Soviet political prisoners who preferred to be imprisoned in the gulags to being free. In the gulags they could express their political beliefs at will, with no fear of being treated worse than they already were being treated. In society at large, however, were they to express their beliefs they would be returned to the gulags, or face similar punishment—and, being free, they would be tempted to betray their deeply held beliefs to avoid that.[34]

It is important to note that the conclusion that has now been reached— that fewer choices might indeed be preferable to less, from the point of view of a valuer of autonomy—has been reached *not* by asking the question of whether agents *in general* would be better able to exercise their autonomy were this particular option (e.g., to sell a kidney) to be eliminated from their choice-sets but by asking the question of whether *a particular agent* would be better served with respect to her exercise of autonomy by having a certain choice-set that contains a smaller number of options than an alternative. This point is important, for it shows that the scope of this argument in favor of the claim that a valuer of autonomy should prefer persons to have fewer choices rather than more is more limited than that of the standard arguments discussed previously. This is because the individualistic basis of this argument precludes it from being used to support a blanket assertion that persons *in general* would be able to exercise their autonomy more effectively were they to be precluded from choosing certain particular options. Unlike the standard arguments discussed previously, then, this argument in favor of the view that a valuer of autonomy should prefer that (some) persons have fewer choices rather than more cannot be used to support any particular policy proposals concerning the prohibition of certain options (such as, for example, the option to sell a kidney by a live vendor, or to be a paid subject for medical research) for, unlike those arguments, it does not operate at a sufficiently general level to establish this. Thus, the mere fact that a valuer of autonomy should accept that fewer choices can be preferable to more does not show that any particular options should be removed from the choice-set that is available to persons in general.[35]

## CONCLUSION

It has been argued in this chapter that although the standard arguments in favor of the claim that, from the point of view of a person who values autonomy, a person's having fewer choices could be preferable to her having more are mistaken, it is still right to hold that for *some* persons this claim is still correct. Given a person's particular motivational-set, she could exercise her autonomy more effectively were she to have a set of options available to her that had a smaller number of elements than some alternative-sets. Unlike the standard arguments that are offered to support the claim that a valuer of autonomy should prefer that persons have fewer options rather than more, however, this conclusion cannot be used to support any particular policy proposals, for it does not operate at a sufficient level of generality to do so. In particular, it cannot be used to support any policy proposals concerning bioethical issues (such as, for example, the sale of human organs) that are based upon restricting persons choice-sets out of concern for their autonomy. Yet although the arguments in this chapter concerning the relationship between autonomy and choice cannot be used to support arguments that are offered at the level of public policy, they do show that a person's having a restricted number of options from which to choose is not necessarily incompatible with her being able to exercise her autonomy to a maximally effective degree. (Indeed, certain restrictions might actually serve to *enhance* her ability to do so.) This issue of the relationship between autonomy and constraint will be the subject of the next chapter.

# 7  Autonomy and Constraint

## INTRODUCTION

The arguments in the last chapter led to the conclusion that, from the point of view of a defender of autonomy, a person's having more choices is (generally) better than her having fewer. This conclusion would seem to imply that a person's being subject to constraints would serve to compromise her autonomy, insofar as such constraints would result in her having fewer choices available to her. However, a person's being subject to constraints is not only compatible with her being able fully to exercise her autonomy, but being subject to constraint is a condition of her being able to be autonomous at all. This point is not, however, of only parochial interest to autonomy theorists. This is because, as will be noted below, the discussion over the degree to which persons must be constrained to be autonomous is parallel to discussions in bioethics concerning the status of ethical decision-making in situations in which there is no recognized objective morality.[1] To argue for the conclusion that persons need to be subject to constraints to be autonomous what might be termed an "extreme voluntarist" (or neo-existentialist) approach to autonomy will be examined, according to which a person is most autonomous if she is free from all constraints. It will be argued that this position is incoherent. Insofar as a person's exercise of her autonomy requires that she guide and direct her actions in accordance with her own desires and values and that these be authoritative for her, then a person whose choices are unconstrained by such desires and values cannot exercise autonomy at all.

That a person's being subject to *internal* constraints upon her choices and actions is not only compatible with, but required by, her being able fully to exercise her autonomy does not show, however, that her being subject to *external* constraints (such as those imposed by her economic circumstances) is also compatible with her fully exercising her autonomy. (This, of course, has implications for debates in bioethics, such as those concerning kidney sales or paying research subjects, which address issues relating to the morality of incentives.) To begin to show that the imposition of such constraints can be fully compatible with a person's fully exercising her autonomy the case of self-imposed commitment will be considered. It will be argued that the imposition of constraints designed to ensure that the person in question adheres to her commitments are similar in kind to those that persons' value-sets impose upon them, and, as such, do not compromise the exercise of autonomy by the persons upon whom they are imposed. With this conclusion in hand it will then be argued that certain constraints that persons are *involuntarily* subject to also fail to compromise their exercise of their autonomy—and that this is so even if they would strongly prefer *not* to be subject to them. Finally, this chapter will conclude by showing how its conclusion (that a person might not suffer from compromised autonomy even if she is subject to constraints that she would prefer not to be subject to) is compatible with the conclusion of the last chapter (that, from the point of view of view of a defender of autonomy, a person's having more choices is better than her having fewer).

## UNCHOSEN CONSTRAINTS

### Against Extreme Voluntarism

At the end of the last chapter it was concluded that, from the point of view of a defender of autonomy, a person's having more choices is (generally) better for her than having fewer. Taking this conclusion further, it might appear that a person's being able to choose anything, and so having no constraints imposed upon her choices at all, would, from the point of view of a valuer of autonomy, be the most desirable situation for her to be in. Such a situation is described by Frankfurt:

> Now suppose that someone is in a position to select from a field of alternatives that has not merely been expanded but has no boundaries at all. Suppose, in other words, that every conceivable course of action is both available and eligible for choice. If the limits of choice have genuinely been wiped out, some possible courses of action will affect the person's desires and preferences themselves and hence bring about profound changes in his volitional character. It will be possible, then, for him to change those aspects of his nature that determine what choices he makes. He will be in a position to redesign his own will.[2]

On the face of it, such radical freedom might seem appealing to a defender of autonomy. After all, if, from the point of view of such a person, a person's having more choices is better for her than her having fewer, her having the maximum number of choices that is conceptually possible would be the best situation to be in. But the appeal that such radical freedom seems to have for a valuer of autonomy is not only illusory: it is incoherent. To see this, it should first be noted that for a person's choices to be normative for him he must have some reason for making them. This claim need not commit one to the view that a person's choices are normative for him only if he has some particular reason in mind for making them when he does so. A person who acts spontaneously but who can *ex post facto* offer non-*ad hoc* justifications for his actions will still be acting for reasons. A person who redesigns his substantial (i.e., constitutive) will for himself through making radically free choices, however, will lack any reason for preferring one course of action over another, and so *none* of his choices will be normative for him. In constructing his will *de novo* through making a radically free choice such a person would have had to have been entirely unbounded with respect to what will he could choose. He would thus have no reason to choose one will over another. The will that he does choose, then, will be one that he has no reason to adopt as his own. But, since this is so, even though this will might itself subsequently appear to give him reasons for action it will always be open to him to question why he should care about such normativity. This is because he had no reason for choosing the will that appears to provide such normativity to him. He thus has no reason for accepting the apparent normativity drawn from that will, over that which he could draw (albeit equally apparently) from another. A radically free agent, then, might be radically free, but he would lack all self-direction, and hence all autonomy, for he would have no *self* to guide his *self*-direction.[3]

Perhaps, however, this argument against the extreme voluntarist is too strong and proves too much. This argument is based on the claim that if a person merely picks an aspect of his preference structure to be his own it will give him no reason in itself to choose one thing over another in the future, since his original picking of that aspect of preference structure could not in itself render its judgments normative for him. However, a proponent of the extreme voluntarist position could respond by claiming that if a person's merely picking to adopt a particular preference structure for no reason precludes it from giving him any reason to act one way rather than another in the future, then a person who is ambivalent about endorsing a particular preference structure that he has and so has to just pick whether to endorse it would also be precluded from subsequently having a preference structure that provides him with reasons to act.[4] However, the extreme voluntarist might continue, it is typically not thought that ambivalence leads to a person's subsequently not having reasons for action when he acts on the preferences that he arbitrarily endorsed. Since this is so, then, it seems that we should not assume that when a person constructs a will for himself through radical choice this will undermine the possibility of his having reasons for his future actions.

This possible response by the extreme voluntarist is plausible—but there are important disanalogies between pickings made in situations when a person is ambivalent towards an aspect of his preference structure and the making of a radical choice that should lead one to reject it. When a person is ambivalent between endorsing or rejecting an aspect of his preference structure that he has, he will be in a situation whereby his motivational-set gives him equally good reasons both to accept it and reject it, and so he just has to pick whether to do so or not. However, this does not mean that this aspect of his motivational-set would not give him reasons to act subsequent to its (arbitrary) endorsement. Prior to his recognizing that he was ambivalent towards it this aspect of his preference structure did give him reasons to act—and these reasons were not dependent upon his own (Hobbesian) will.[5] In picking to endorse aspects of his preference structure, then, this person was picking to *continue* to be bound by the reasons that it gave him. Unlike the reasons that a will that is the construct of a radical choice is purported (i.e., by extreme voluntarists) to impose upon a person, then, the reasons that would be imposed upon him by aspects of his preference structure that he picked to retain after being ambivalent towards it would not be entirely dependent upon his will, for they would have applied to him *prior to* his picking them. Although a person who picks to endorse aspects of his preference structure to resolve ambivalence would partially constitute himself in so doing, he would not be doing so *de novo*, and the reasons given by the preference structure that he picked would be supported by other aspects of his preference structure that he did not pick. Thus, it is not his endorsement alone that makes the reasons that flow from the aspect of his preference structure that he picks to endorse normative for him, as is the case with will constituted through radical choice. Rather, it is his endorsement of it *together with* its history of independently supplying him with reasons for action.

Yet this reply to the previous extreme voluntarist response leads us only to another possible defense of the extreme voluntarist position. This reply rests on the claim that a person's arbitrarily picked preference structure would give him reasons for action *provided that* it gave him reasons for action prior to his picking it to do so. However, the extreme voluntarist might rejoin, this response is not applicable in all cases in which a person picks to be motivated by one preference structure rather than another in a situation when neither had previously given him reason to act. Consider, for example, a football fan who moves to a new location and who arbitrarily picks which one of two local football teams he will support, without having any reason for endorsing either one over the other. (Their players are equivalent in skill and charisma, their grounds are equivalent, their supporters are all equally violent, and so on.) Yet once this person has picked Manchester United rather than Manchester City to be the team that he supports, that he is a United supporter is not irrelevant to him when he makes his future football-orientated choices.[6]

It will not suffice as a rejoinder to this extreme voluntarist reply to note that this person already had reason to support a football team, for his preference to be a football fan is not at issue. Rather, what is at issue is the apparent fact that, after he picked United, he had reason to support them over City (i.e., he has reason to be a *United supporter* rather than just a *football fan*), and that *this* reason was completely lacking prior to his picking to support United. It seems, then, that this extreme voluntarist reply does show that a person's picking one preference structure over another can alone endow it with normativitity vis-à-vis his future choices. And, as such, it seems that it shows that the extreme voluntarist position is a coherent one—and that a valuer of autonomy should (generally) prefer a person's (initial) choice-set to be unbounded.

Yet to accept the extreme voluntarist position on this basis would be too hasty, for another objection can be leveled against this position. It was noted previously that there is an important disanalogy between pickings made in situations of ambivalence towards one's preference structure and instances of radical choice. This is that in the former case it is not the person's endorsement *alone* that renders his preference structure authoritative for him, but his endorsement of it *together with* the fact that prior to his endorsement of it, it was authoritative for him. That is, a person's endorsement of a preference structure does not alone endow it with the authority to give him reasons for action, but it is this endorsement *together with something else that is not under his control* that endows his preferences with such authority for him. The same point can be made here. This last defense of extreme voluntarism rests on the plausible view that a person could have reasons for supporting one football team over another even though he merely arbitrarily picked which team to support. The plausibility of this view, however, depends on our taking a longitudinal view of this person's support of his team, rather than a punctuated one. That is, it is plausible to think that a person who merely picked to support United over City thirty years ago would now have reasons to orientate his football-related activities around his support of United, even though his original choice of them as "his" team was an arbitrary one. It is not, however, so plausible to think that a person who had picked United as "his" team ten seconds ago would have similar reasons to orientate his football-related activities around his support of them. Put simply, whereas it would likely come as a surprise to us to hear that a thirty-year supporter of United had suddenly decided to support City (and we would think that he would have had to have had good reasons for so doing), it would not surprise us much to hear that a ten-second supporter of United had changed his allegiance to City (and we would not think that he would similarly have had to have had good reasons for doing so). But that the plausibility of this defense of the extreme voluntarist view rests on our taking a longitudinal view of this fan's support of "his" team rather than a punctuated one indicates that it is not his picking of which team that he should support *alone* that provides him with reasons for support—it is this picking *together with something else*: here, the length of time that he has been a United supporter. This is unsurprising, for when persons invest emotionally in projects such as the support of a football team their involvement in such projects itself provides them with reasons for action as they come to identify themselves with these projects.[7]

It is important to note that it is the person's involvement in the project in question rather than his mere association with it that gives him reasons for action. To give him reasons for action the project in question must be one that has become part of his self-identity, even if his involvement with it began with his merely picking to be associated with it. Thus, even though the previously mentioned football fan might have originally picked United to support merely to satisfy his desire to be a supporter of a team, as his support of United continues he might come adopt the attitudes of a United supporter, and so come to value the team for its own sake. Even though the originating cause of his support for United would have been his picking United to support, the sustaining cause of his support would be facts both about the team, and about himself as a United supporter. As such, then, it is not the picking of United that gives the fan reasons to direct himself in one way rather than another so much as it is his picking of United together with the fact that this led to him *becoming a supporter of United*, where his becoming a supporter of United was not under his direct control. Since this is so, then, the prior defense of the extreme voluntarist view fails, since it must rest on the claim that it is the fan's picking United alone that gives him reasons to orientate his football-based activities in a certain way.

There is, however, one final argument that is available to the extreme voluntarist: that if a person can over time come to identify herself with certain preferences, and so the preferences that she picked will come to give her reasons for action, then would it not be better from the point of view of a valuer of autonomy for persons to be subject to no constraints, so that they could choose their own preference structures, which could, in time, provide them with reasons for action? Again, however, this argument in favor of the extreme voluntarist position is mistaken. This is because the proponent of this argument assumes that, from the point of view of a valuer of autonomy, it would be better for persons to pick their preference structures, on the grounds then they could be autonomous not only with respect to their desires and actions that flow from these preference structures but also with respect to their picking of the preference structures themselves. Yet while it is true that persons who picked their preference structures in this way could, in the way outlined previously, come to be autonomous with respect to the desires and actions that flowed from them they would not be autonomous with respect to their initial picking of their preference structures, for then they would lack selves to direct such pickings. From the point of view of a valuer of autonomy, then, it would not matter whether persons constituted themselves *de novo* in this way, or whether their preference structures were given to them, for in neither case would the persons concerned be autonomous with respect to their preference structures, although they might be with respect to the desires and actions that flowed from them. Moreover, were she to offer this argument the extreme voluntarist would have to concede that, from the point of a view of a valuer of autonomy, it is not the case that a person's being free from constraint would be better than her being subject to it. This is because in offering this argument the extreme voluntarist would be conceding that a person's coming to be constrained by the boundaries of his preference structure is necessary for him to be able to exercise autonomy—and hence that, from the point of view of a valuer of autonomy, a person's being subject to fewer constraints is not necessarily better than her being subject to more.

## Volitional Necessity and Unthinkability

This rejection of the extreme voluntarist view of the relationship between autonomy and constraint leads to two further questions: how bounded must persons be by their preference structures to be autonomous, and how can autonomy arise from preference structures that are themselves held heteronomously?

The simple answers to these questions are: sufficiently and readily.[8] These answers are not, however, as inconsequential as they might seem. To address the first of these questions, one should first consider Frankfurt's views on the relationship between autonomy and the constraints that are imposed upon a person by her volitional nature. For Frankfurt, "An autonomous agent is, by definition, governed by himself alone. He acts entirely under his own control. It seems natural and reasonable to presume that when a person is acting under his own control, he will guide his conduct with an eye to those things that he considers to be of greatest importance to him."[9] For Frankfurt, then, "A person acts autonomously only when his volitions derive from the essential character of his will."[10] To elaborate on this, it must be recognized that, for Frankfurt, the "essence" of a thing consists of "those characteristics without which it cannot be what it is," and so "the essential nature of a person is constituted by his necessary personal characteristics."[11] These "necessary personal characteristics" are "characteristics of his will," which are "reflexive, or higher-order, volitional features" of it.[12] For Frankfurt, these features of a person's will that comprise its essence are those that determine for the person concerned the limits of what he can will to do. The first of these features concerns what he cannot bring himself to do; this is the requirement that a person refrain from performing an action because it is unthinkable for him. To be a genuine instance of unthinkability in the sense that the unthinkability of the act in question is one that is (at least partially) constitutive of the essence of the (substantial) will of the person concerned, she must not only find the act in question unthinkable in the sense that she could not will to do it, but that "acting with an intention to make the unthinkable thinkable is itself something that the person cannot bring himself to do."[13] When all courses of action but one are unthinkable for a person he is constrained by volitional necessity. To illustrate this Frankfurt offers the example of Martin Luther, when he stated "Here I stand; *I can do no other.*"[14] Luther could neither bring himself to do anything other than what he did, nor could he have taken steps to render one of the alternative courses of action that were in his power to perform thinkable for him. For Frankfurt, then, a person will only act autonomously "when his volitions derive from the essential nature of his will," and since, for Frankfurt, "the essential nature of a person consists of what he must will," a person will only act autonomously when he is volitionally necessitated to do so, or when his refraining from performing a certain action stems from its unthinkability.[15] According to Frankfurt, then, persons must be very strictly bounded by their preference structures if they are to be autonomous with respect to their actions. Indeed, for Frankfurt, a person will be autonomous with respect to her actions only if all other courses of action were unthinkable for her.[16]

How plausible is Frankfurt's account of autonomy? In "Autonomy, Necessity, and Love" Frankfurt noted that, for Kant, "The autonomous will can only be one that incorporates what Kant calls a 'pure' will. It must conform, in other words, to the requirements of a will that is indifferent to all personal interests. . ."[17] However, noted Frankfurt, "this pure will is a very peculiar and unlikely place in which to locate an indispensable condition of personal autonomy."[18] In this Frankfurt is undoubtedly correct—but precisely the same criticism could be leveled at his own (stringent) account of personal autonomy. To see this, consider the example of Lord Fawn, which Frankfurt uses to illustrate the concept of unthinkability. Fawn had invited his estate steward, Andy Gowran, to testify to him that he had seen his, Fawn's, fiancée embracing another man. Yet although he had resolved to ask Gowran about the actions of his fiancée, Fawn found that it was unthinkable for him "to share a matter of such intimate concern with a person so inferior to himself in breeding and class."[19] For Frankfurt, then, none of the actions that Fawn performed that led up to the moment when continuing to converse with Gowran for him were actions that he was autonomous with respect to, for it was only the act of refraining from continuing the conversation with Gowran that stemmed from "the essential nature of his will," owing to its unthinkability. But this is a "very peculiar and unlikely" view of the scope of Fawn's autonomy. Instead, it seems far more plausible that (to draw on the account of practical autonomy that was developed in Chapter 1) insofar as it was Fawn, and not someone else, who was directing the actions that Fawn performed that led up to the moment when he found himself unable to continue conversing with Gowran, and insofar as Fawn decided to perform these actions in accordance with a decision procedure that he endorsed, that he was autonomous with respect to them. Like Kant's, then, Frankfurt's account of autonomy is far too rarefied.[20]

Is it possible, then, to steer a middle course between the Charybdis of the unbounded selves posited by the extreme voluntarists, and the Scylla of the tightly bounded self that Frankfurt envisages, that will exercise autonomy only very rarely? Frankfurt seems to think that it is not—that these are our only two options. This is because, according to Frankfurt, a person must have "inviolable boundaries"; he must have ideals, or limits, that he "cannot bring himself to betray."[21] Were a person to lack such ideals, claims Frankfurt, "nothing is unthinkable for him; there are no limits to what he might be willing to do. He can make whatever decisions he likes and shape his will just as he pleases."[22] Indeed, such a person's "will is anarchic, moved by mere impulse and inclination."[23] But there is no reason to share Frankfurt's pessimism here. To see this, consider the character of Conway in Theodore Sturgeon's short story "The Dark Room."[24] Conway occasionally attended parties given by his friend Beck. At each party one of the guests would find himself or herself humiliated by performing actions that were utterly out of character; a faithful wife would find herself in bed with the husband of her best friend, for example, or a lady novelist who wrote children's stories would regale the company with an obscene story. Curious as to the source of these incidents, Conway breaks into Beck's house to discover that it was inhabited by an alien. The alien explains to him that he feeds on human humiliation and satisfies his need for this through arranging these events to occur at Beck's parties. Conway is curious as to why he has never been humiliated at Beck's parties and learns that he is "immune": there is nothing that he would not do; there is nothing that is unthinkable for him. Yet, despite Conway's potential willingness to do anything, he does not have a merely anarchic will, "moved by mere impulse and inclination." Instead, he has a stable and consistent set of preferences that enable him to plan and order his actions and to make choices accordingly. As such, Conway avoids the Charybdis of extreme voluntarism. Moreover, Conway is not (necessarily) a mere (nonautonomous) wanton, but, instead, could be aware of the decision procedures that he uses when deliberating what to do and accepts them as his own. Conway, then, could satisfy the conditions for personal autonomy that were outlined in Chapter 1. He thus avoids the Scylla of Frankfurt's tightly bounded self. In answer to the first of the two questions previously, then, Conway is *sufficiently constrained* by his stable preference structure to be able to exercise autonomy.

But this answer to that question might strike both the extreme voluntarist and Frankfurt as being unsatisfying. After all, they might both object, in merely having a stable preference structure Conway is not really constrained at all. In being unfettered by having a determinate substantial will he could, they might both observe, simply chose to reform his preference structure at will, for he is not bound by having an essential nature. This observation is correct—but it lacks the force that its proponents might believe it possesses. While it is true that Conway could choose to reform his preference structure *de novo* (although he would not only have no reason to do so but would have no reason to choose any particular alternate structure) he is, like the longtime United supporter in the example given previously, invested in the structure that he has. As such he would not revise his preference structure since this would be too costly. Thus, even though he is not constrained by having a will with an essential nature, the range of options that are reasonable for him to pursue is constrained by his actual preference structure. To hold that Conway is constrained in this way is compatible with claiming that there is nothing that he would not do, for given the right conditions he would do anything. The claim here is merely that not every option is a live one for him at every time, and so even though he is not subject to the sort of logical or conceptual constraints that Frankfurt believes are required for autonomy, Conway is subject to constraint—and subject in a way that is sufficient for him to be autonomous.

## Autonomy and Contingent Preferences

With this answer to the first of the previous two questions in place, it is time to turn to the second: How can autonomy arise from preference structures that are themselves held heteronomously?

In the previous response to the extreme voluntarist it was argued that to be able to exercise autonomy a person must be able to choose on the basis of a stable preference structure, where the reason-giving authority of this preference structure could not stem solely from the fact that he chose it. As such, then, a person's exercise of autonomy must be grounded on facts about him that he was not autonomous with respect to. On the face of it this might seem puzzling. An autonomous person is widely held to be one who "is under his or her own control, master of his or her own destiny."[25] If, however, autonomy requires that a person act on the basis of facts about himself or herself that she is not in control of, not master of, then it seems that no-one could ever be autonomous. Autonomy, it seems, is thus a self-defeating concept, for the conditions that must be met for a person to exercise it would themselves defeat this very possibility.

If this bleak conclusion is not to be accepted, one of two options must be chosen. The first is to side with the extreme voluntarist and to hold that the exercise of autonomy must be based on a preference structure that the person in question has chosen for herself. To pursue this line of argument would, however, require not just the abandonment of the line of argument that was offered previously against the extreme voluntarist position but also its refutation. The second option is to reject the view that an autonomous person must be motivated to act by a preference structure that he is autonomous with respect to. Given the strength of the previous responses to the extreme voluntarist position the second of these options is the more attractive of the two. But even so, this does not mean that it will be an easy option to pursue, for the weight of philosophical opinion seems to be ranged against it. Marilyn Friedman, for example, writes of "the old adage that like comes from like; autonomy is not expected to emerge out of processes which are not autonomous, not a person's 'own' to begin with."[26] Similarly, Stefaan Cuypers asks, "How can there be autonomy without autonomous foundations?"[27] Finally, and perhaps most influentially, Christman outlines this problem (which he dubs the "*Ab Initio* Problem") in the form of a question that the proponents of any analysis of autonomy must answer: "[H]ow can a desire be autonomous if it was formed or evaluated by a process that was not *itself* autonomous"?[28]

To answer the questions posed by Cuypers and Christman, and hence to dissolve the *Ab Initio* Problem, the underlying intuition that supports it should be examined more closely. This is the same intuition that underlay the extreme voluntarist's claim that a person enjoys maximal autonomy when she is free of all constraint: that, to be autonomous with respect to an action a person must control all of the elements that are internal to him (including his desires, preferences, values, and so on) that led him to perform that act. It might be tempting at this point to fall back on the arguments outlined previously, and to claim that insofar as taking this intuition seriously leads to an incoherent position it should be rejected. But this would be a mistake. To do so would be to fail to show where the adherents of intuition go astray in accepting it, a task that is more foundational than that of showing why accepting this intuition will lead one into an incoherent position. And the adherents of this intuition go astray in two related ways: in misunderstanding what autonomy is a property of and (and as a result of this) of misunderstanding the relationship between persons and their preference structures.[29]

Let us take each of these mistakes in turn. It is natural to accept the *Ab Initio* Problem as a genuine problem for theories of autonomy if one assumes that autonomy is a property of a person's psychological states or processes.[30] As was argued in Chapter 1, however, this is mistaken; autonomy is *not* a property of a person's psychological states or processes (or actions), but a property of *persons with respect to* their psychological states or processes (or actions). This is an important distinction, for it shows that one cannot ask whether something is autonomous simpliciter, but, instead, that one must ask whether a person, P, is autonomous with respect to some state or action S. That is, it shows that the ascription of autonomy is a two-place relation ("P is autonomous with respect to S") and not merely a one-place relation ("S is autonomous").[31] Once this is recognized, one should also recognize that the scope of the question of whether a person P is autonomous with respect to something S can only be asked of S's that are *separable* from the P in question. Thus, if some S is not separable from some P, one cannot ask whether P is autonomous with respect to S, for the necessary two-place relationship between P and S that is necessary for this question to be applicable will not exist.[32] Recognizing this first mistake on the part of the adherents of this intuition leads to the recognition of the second. Given that the ascription of autonomy is a two-place relation, to ask whether a person is autonomous with respect to his preference structure is to assume that persons and their preference structures are separable; that is, persons could exist apart from their preference structures. But, unless one adopts a strict (and implausible) bodily criterion of personal identity, this assumption is unfounded, for persons are in some way constituted by their stable and cross-temporal psychological states. The answer to the question of exactly how persons are constituted by their stable and cross-temporal psychological states (that is, the answer to the problem of personal identity) is, however, orthogonal to the issue at hand here.[33] Instead, the important point is that insofar as persons are at least partially constituted by such psychological states—which will include their stable preference structures—the question of whether they are autonomous with respect to those that are constitutive of them cannot arise.

The *Ab Initio* Problem, then, readily dissolves once it is recognized that it is based upon two mistaken assumptions. And this should come as no surprise given the account of practical autonomy that was developed in Chapter 1. On this account, recall, it is necessary for a person P to be autonomous with respect to a decision D that she makes that the information on which she based the decision has not been affected by another agent with the end of leading her to make a particular decision, or a decision from a particular class of decisions (or if it has been, then she is aware of the way in which it has been so affected, while if she is not aware of its being so affected when it has been then she did not make the decision that the agent who was affecting the information she had access to with the intent of leading her to make a particular decision intended her to make), where the maximum degree to which a person will be autonomous with respect to a decision that she makes will be determined by the degree to which it is the result of a decision procedure that she is satisfied with as being her decision procedure for making the type of the decision that is in question.[34] Or, more briefly and prosaically (if less accurately) a person P is autonomous with respect to a decision D that she makes if it is she, and not another agent, A, who controls her making of D. As such, recall, the account of practical autonomy that has been developed and defended in this volume is a *political* account of autonomy, such that the question of whether P is autonomous with respect to D is decided by examining whether the outcome of P's critical reflection that led to her making D was subject to the control of others. Given this, a person could be fully autonomous with respect to her decisions even if her making of them was based upon elements of her preference structure that she had not critically evaluated, provided that the critical evaluation that she did engage in and that issued in her decisions was free from external control. Contra Berofsky, then, the mere fact that persons have contingent preference-sets is no bar to their being "as autonomous as we can easily imagine them to be."[35] Autonomy is thus not merely "an intelligible ideal that all of us approximate only to a certain degree" but a live possibility for normal adult humans.[36]

## Economic Constraints

The unchosen constraints that are imposed upon persons by their preference structures, then, are thus not only not inimical to the exercise of their autonomy but (given the arguments against the extreme voluntarist position, previously) required for this. The same, however, cannot be said for constraints that are imposed upon persons by virtue of their economic impoverishment. Like the acceptance of the *Ab Initio* Problem as a genuine problem for autonomy theorists, the view that poverty typically compromises personal autonomy is widespread.[37] Indeed, it often features as a foundational assumption in arguments within bioethics that are developed to show that concern for autonomy cannot support offering impoverished persons incentives to perform actions that they would not otherwise perform (such as sell their organs or participate in clinical trials), on the grounds that such persons' autonomy has already been compromised by their poverty, and so they cannot autonomously consent to such offers were they to be made to them.[38] It is not difficult to see the appeal of this position. After all, if a person lives in Dickensian poverty, working in a blacking factory for eighteen hours a day, seven days a week, earning enough merely to feed herself a starvation diet, it seems that her opportunities for exercising her autonomy are limited (given the plausible assumption that this is not how she would chose to spend her life were other options to be available to her). The view that impoverished persons suffer from compromised autonomy has been famously (although indirectly) argued for by Joseph Raz through his example of the Man in the Pit. This man must spend his life interred in a pit, with his choices limited to "whether to eat now or a little later, whether to sleep now or a little later, whether to scratch his left ear or not."[39] Raz argues that the Man in the Pit fails to enjoy an autonomous life for he does not have "an adequate range of options to choose from," for the only options that he has are trivial ones.[40] The same points could also be made with respect to persons who live in poverty.

Yet despite the initial plausibility of the view that economic impoverishment would typically compromise the autonomy of persons subject to it this claim should not be too readily accepted. Simply because a person is economically impoverished does not mean that she is any less autonomous simpliciter than someone who is not, for she need not be any less able to exercise her autonomy than her wealthier counterpart.[41] An impoverished person can still make her own choices and decisions on the basis of her own values, and she can still assess her own decision-making procedure to see whether it is one that she is satisfied with.[42] Even an impoverished person, then, would still be able to exercise her autonomy; even the Man in the Pit can still choose when to eat, when to sleep, whether to scratch his ear or not, as well as "how to respond attitudinally to his fate," for "he retains the choice of what to think, what to feel, whether or not to pray."[43] Yet although it is true that even an impoverished person can still exercise her autonomy, as was noted in the previous chapter, the instrumental value of such exercise for her is likely to be low, for she is unlikely to be able to exercise her autonomy as she would wish to do so. Thus, while being subject to economic constraint will not render a person less autonomous than another person who is not subject to such constraint, it will be likely to render her autonomy less instrumentally valuable to her. And, since this is so, if impoverished persons are made (what are to them) attractive offers (such as two million dollars for one of their kidneys, to reprise Cherry's example) it would seem that, *ceteris paribus*, were they to accept such offers they would be able to increase the future instrumental value of their autonomy.[44] Such offers, then, should be welcomed, rather than opposed, by persons who value autonomy.

## Biological Constraints

Just as being subject to economic constraints will be likely to compromise the instrumental value of a person's autonomy to her, so too might her subjection to biological constraints. A biological constraint is a constraint that is imposed upon persons in virtue of their being the type of beings that they are.[45] The inability to fly like a bird, for example, is a biological constraint of this sort, as is the inability to swim underwater like a fish. If a person wished to perform these activities he would be precluded from doing so, and so the instrumental value of his autonomy would be diminished for him. However, like economic constraints, being subject to a particular biological constraint (e.g., the inability to run a four-minute mile) will not render the person subject to it less autonomous simpliciter than another person who is not. It might appear that the instrumental value of the autonomy of only a few persons would be compromised by such biological constraints, for they seem likely to thwart the desires of only a few people. But this appearance is misleading, for biological constraints are imposed upon persons in virtue of their unavoidable aging and eventual death. As such, persons are constrained insofar as they cannot pursue all the options that they might wish to pursue, for their aging and eventual death precludes this.[46] A person cannot, for example, be both an internationally renowned mathematician and an Olympic-standard tennis player even if she were capable of excelling in both fields, for each of these goals requires a degree of dedication during the same period of a person's life that would preclude the pursuit of the other. For the same reason a woman might be precluded from achieving both her goal of having a successful career and her goal of having several children. In general, then, insofar as persons are biologically finite beings their making of choices is likely to preclude them from pursuing other goals and interests that they desire to pursue. A person's biological nature, then, is likely to serve to compromise the instrumental value of their autonomy for him, although it will not render him less able to exercise his autonomy.

## CHOSEN CONSTRAINTS

The type of constraints that have been considered previously have all been *unchosen* constraints; they have all been constraints that have been imposed upon persons without their consent. Since being subject to unchosen constraints not only fails to compromise the ability of a person to exercise her autonomy (although they might compromise its instrumental value for her) but is a prerequisite for this, it is plausible that a person's choosing to subject herself to constraint would similarly fail to compromise her exercise of her autonomy. After all, if the unchosen constraints outlined previously fail to compromise a person's exercise of her autonomy, it would seem natural to hold that the constraints that a person autonomously chooses for herself (and that thus reflect her own desires and values), would similarly fail to compromise her exercise of her autonomy. However, one should not rush to endorse the view that the constraints that a person chooses to be subject to fail to compromise her autonomy. This is because there are three main types of constraints that a person might choose to be subject to; constraints that a person chooses to be subject to, to ensure that she will not pursue a constraining option, constraints that a person imposes upon herself as part of the expression of her values, and constraints that a person chooses to accept that involve her ceding control over her actions to another person.

As was argued in the previous chapter, since the first type of such self-chosen constraints would increase the number of live options that a person would have available to her they would be likely to enhance the instrumental value of her autonomy for her (although, as was also noted in the previous chapter, they would not enhance her ability to exercise her autonomy simpliciter). Such constraints, then, would not compromise the autonomy of the persons who are subject to them. It is the second type of self-chosen constraint, however—constraints that a person imposes upon herself to express her values—that has attracted the greatest degree of philosophical attention. It is this type of constraint that Carolyn M. Stone is writing of when she asks "Is it possible to love another person, or indeed several persons, and still maintain one's autonomy?" Stone's answer is that it is not, since "the autonomous person would preserve a degree of distance from all such emotional attachments. Any attachments formed would have a somewhat provisional nature and be constantly subject to critical scrutiny and review."[47] A similar argument for the incompatibility of self-chosen constraints (such as making a commitment to another person or a particular community) has been considered by Allen Buchanan:

> Community requires commitment, but commitment is not an attachment one can simply freely choose to sever. Any attachment that one freely chooses, one can freely choose to sever. For liberal man all attachments are freely chosen. Therefore, liberal man is incapable of commitment, and, being incapable of commitment, is barred from community.[48]

Putting this argument in terms of autonomy and commitment the argument is that autonomy and the constraints of commitment are logically incompatible because all of the commitments that an autonomous person would make would be ones that she could freely sever. Since being committed to a community is not an attachment that a person can freely sever, it is not a commitment that could be made by an autonomous person. Thus, a person cannot be both autonomous and committed to a community.[49]

Although this argument, and that offered by Stone, for the view that autonomy is incompatible with self-chosen commitments are both initially plausible, they should be rejected. As Buchanan notes, the argument that he considers for this view is flawed in that it is simply not true that "Any attachment that one freely chooses, one can freely choose to sever." A person might, for example, freely choose to enter into a slavery contract that has been specifically designed to prohibit her from having any exit from the enslavement in question. There is also another, more general, argument that can be leveled against the view that autonomy and self-chosen (and irrevocable) commitments are incompatible with each other. A person who commits himself to another (e.g., through marriage), or to an ideal (e.g., to serve his country, right or wrong), or to a way of life (e.g., as a member of the sex opposite to that which he was physically born as) will do so because he believes that such commitment would better enable him (or even simply enable him) to achieve his goals or to realize his values.[50] When a person autonomously enters into such a commitment, then, he will be acting in a way that is likely to enhance the instrumental value of his autonomy. Furthermore, his entering into such a commitment does not render him less autonomous simpliciter, for it does not render him less able to guide and direct himself in accordance with his own desires and values. As such, then, from the point of view of a defender of autonomy it is desirable, not lamentable, that persons with particular preference structures (i.e., those that would be satisfied through such commitments) can enter into such commitments. Thus, not only should the possibility of (for example) irrevocable marriages be praised, but so, too, should persons who value autonomy favor the possibility of persons pursuing certain irrevocable medical procedures, such as sterilization, sex changes, or cosmetic surgery—no matter how radical the latter might be.

One might, however, object that this presents a rather rosy picture of commitments such as marriage, service to one's country, or even to certain ways of life—such as a transgendered man's commitment to live as a woman. What, such a skeptic might ask, of the person who makes a mistake: who makes a commitment to another person, or to his country, or to be another gender that he later comes to regret—and yet which he cannot break? Surely such a person would suffer from compromised autonomy as a result of his self-chosen commitment? This objection certainly serves the useful purpose of highlighting the fact that not all self-chosen commitments will enhance the instrumental value of the autonomy of those who subject themselves to them. However, it does not show that such (unfortunate) commitments would compromise the autonomy of those subject to them simpliciter, for they would still be able to guide and direct their actions in accordance with their own desires and values.[51] Nor does it show that such commitments would necessarily compromise the ability of those subject to them to exercise their autonomy effectively. As such, then, there is no necessary incompatibility between self-chosen commitments and autonomy, whether this latter is understood either in terms of its intrinsic value (autonomy simpliciter) or its instrumental value to its possessor (measured by the degree to which she is able to exercise it effectively in the pursuit of her own desires and values).

What, then, of the third type of self-chosen constraint: those that a person chooses to accept that involve her ceding control over her actions to another person? An example of such a self-chosen constraint might be that of a monk who cedes control over his actions to his abbot, or a soldier who cedes control over his actions to his superior officers. Such self-chosen constraints differ in kind from the two discussed previously, for, unlike those types of constraints, subjecting oneself to these sorts of constraints involves the abdication of control over one's actions to another. Insofar as such abdication would lead to an agent other than the person who has chosen to be constrained in this way directing the actions of the constrainee, subjecting oneself to such constraints will indeed result in the constrainee's autonomy being diminished with respect to the actions that he performs at the behest of his constrainer.[52] However, this does not itself show that a defender of autonomy should oppose persons choosing this third type of self-imposed constraint, for if one holds autonomy to be primarily instrumental (rather than intrinsic) value one should not oppose a person's voluntarily subjecting himself to such constraints in an attempt to achieve something that he values more than the exercise of his autonomy. This, though, will be further discussed in Chapter 10, when the value of autonomy (especially the value of autonomy within the context of contemporary discussions of bioethics) will be considered.

## CONCLUSION

It was argued in this chapter that being subject to constraints, either unchosen or chosen, is not incompatible either with a person's autonomy simpliciter or with her autonomy possessing a maximal degree of instrumental value for her. Indeed, the arguments in this chapter support stronger conclusions than this, for, in criticizing the extreme voluntarist position, they support both the view that a person must be subject to unchosen constraints for her to be autonomous at all, and that the ability to subject oneself to chosen constraints will, for certain persons, enhance the instrumental value of their autonomy to them.

These conclusions are not, however, incompatible with those reached in the last chapter, where it was argued that, from the point of view of a defender of autonomy, a person's having more choices is (typically) preferable to her having fewer. The reason for this should be clear from the concluding discussion of that chapter: that what matters from the point of view of a defender of autonomy is not how many choices a person might have but whether the choices that she has access to are those that she would wish to pursue. As such, then, a valuer of autonomy should not be concerned about the imposition of constraints upon persons *per se*, but, rather, with the question of whether those constraints remove from the choice-set of the person so constrained options that she finds appealing—such as, for example, the option to sell a kidney in a current market for such.

# 8 Autonomy, Privacy, and Patient Confidentiality

## INTRODUCTION

Ever since Warren and Brandeis defined the right to privacy as "the right to be let alone," it has been widely held in both the legal and the philosophical literature that a violation of one's privacy will necessarily also compromise one's autonomy.[1] This purported connection between privacy and autonomy is also widely accepted within the bioethics literature, with the protection of the privacy of a patient's medical records frequently being justified on the grounds that this is required by respect for patient autonomy. Sabine Michalowski, for example, notes explicitly that "One justification for the protection of medical confidentiality is based on the premise that it seeks to guarantee respect for a patient's autonomy and privacy when entering a professional relationship with a physician,"[2] while James W. Jones holds that "Confidentiality in the professional relationship is a duty derived from respect for the patient's autonomy."[3] Yet even though the view that respect for patient autonomy requires the protection of the confidentiality of patients' medical records there has been surprisingly few arguments offered in favor of this view. This paucity of argument in the bioethical literature on autonomy and patient confidentiality would be understandable if it had already been established within the philosophical or legal literature at large that a violation of a person's privacy would necessarily serve to compromise her autonomy. It is thus all the more striking that even in this more general literature very few arguments have been offered in support of this generally accepted claim.

The purpose of this chapter, then, is to reexamine the claim that a concern for maintaining patient confidentiality is justified out of respect for patient autonomy. To do so those few arguments that have been offered in defense of the view that a violation of a person's privacy will necessarily fail to compromise her autonomy will be examined—and will be found wanting. This is because, as will be argued below, they either rest on a mischaracterization of privacy or they fail to distinguish between its overt and covert violation. The aim of this chapter, however, is not entirely negative. Once the standard arguments that have been offered in support of the view that a violation of a person's privacy will necessarily compromise her autonomy have been rejected, an argument will be developed that shows there is indeed a connection between the violation of a person's privacy and the compromising of her autonomy. This argument will not, however, show that there is a necessary connection between autonomy and privacy. Instead, it will show that the relationship between privacy and autonomy is merely a contingent one, such that a violation of one's privacy will only result in the compromise of one's autonomy if other conditions are also met. The arguments in this chapter thus have three implications for contemporary discussions of patient confidentiality and autonomy. First, they show that the widely held assumption that a violation of a person's privacy will adversely affect her autonomy is unwarranted. As such, the (initial) arguments in this chapter will provide a *prima facie* reason for believing that one is most justified in being agnostic about whether or not concern for personal autonomy should support concern for patient confidentiality. Second, insofar as the (later) arguments in this chapter will establish that there is a connection between a violation of a person's privacy and the compromise of her autonomy (albeit a contingent one) they will resurrect the view that concern for patient confidentiality can be justified out of respect for patient autonomy. This, however, will appear to provide only cold comfort to persons who believe that the ethical foundation for respect for patient privacy is respect for patient autonomy, for it will transpire that many breaches of patient confidentiality will not serve to compromise the autonomy of those subject to them. Finally, it will be shown that, despite this, a concern for the instrumental value of patient autonomy can ethically justify a concern with patient confidentiality.

The arguments in this chapter, then, will provide a reason for holding that, unless there is reason to believe the contrary, patient confidentiality should not be violated out of respect for patient autonomy. Having noted this one might hold that the arguments in this chapter are moot, insofar as they do not appear to justify a revisionary approach to the question of patient confidentiality. But this would be mistaken for two reasons. First, absent the arguments in this chapter there is an important lacuna in the ethical literature on patient confidentiality. Second—and more importantly—the arguments in this chapter will show that, *contra* received opinion, the concern for patient autonomy provides only an *indirect* justification for concern for patient privacy. And, as will be discussed in Chapter 10, this has important implications for the question of how autonomy is to be valued in contemporary bioethics.

## A PRELIMINARY DISTINCTION

This chapter will address the strong claim that a violation of a person's privacy will *compromise* her autonomy and not the weaker claim that a violation of a person's privacy evinces a *failure to respect* her autonomy. This distinction is important, for it is a simple matter to show that a deliberate violation of a person's privacy might evince a failure to respect her autonomy. A person might fail to respect the autonomy of another in either of two ways. He might fail to take those decisions, or desires, that she is autonomous with respect to into consideration when he is deciding how to act, or he might act so as deliberately to frustrate either the course of action that he believes that she has autonomously decided upon, or those desires that he believes she possesses and is autonomous with respect to. In deliberately violating another's privacy, such a person would seek to gain access to information that he believes that she desires to conceal (such as, for example, her financial records). In seeking to gain access to this information, then, he would either fail to take into account the desire that he believes she has to keep this information private (and so fails to respect her autonomy in the first way) or else he deliberately seeks out this information in order to frustrate her desire to keep this information private (and so fails to respect her autonomy in the second way).

Although it is easy to see how a violation of a person's privacy might evince a failure to respect her autonomy, it is not so clear how a failure to respect a person's privacy will also *compromise* her autonomy.[4] For example, even though James Stewart's character in Hitchcock's *Rear Window* might have failed to respect the autonomy of his neighbors when he spied on them during his convalescence, this mere watching alone did not adversely affect their autonomy simpliciter; it did not compromise their ability to make their own decisions or form their own desires over how they were to behave. And it is this stronger claim that a violation of a person's privacy will compromise her autonomy that is prevalent within the philosophical literature and that forms the basis of much of the bioethical discussion of autonomy and patient confidentiality.[5]

## PRIVACY, AUTONOMY, AND CONTROL

The focus of this chapter, then, is on the robust claim that a violation of a person's privacy will necessarily result in the compromise of her autonomy and not on the weaker claim that a violation of a person's privacy evinces a failure to respect her autonomy. At first sight it seems that there is a simple and elegant way to forge such a necessary connection between a violation of a person's privacy and the compromise of her autonomy. As was argued in Chapter 1, a person suffers from a diminution in his autonomy if the decisions that he makes (and hence the actions that he performs that flow from them) are subject to the control of another. Similarly, it is often argued that a person enjoys privacy with respect to some item of information P if she is able to control others' access to P. Hyman Gross, for example, argues that privacy should be considered "as the condition under which there is control over acquaintance with one's affairs,"[6] while Charles Fried claims that privacy is "the control we have over information about ourselves."[7] This control-based account of privacy also features in discussions of patient confidentiality. For example, Lisa Schwartz, Paul Preece, and Ron Hendry claim that "by helping the patient maintain control over information others have of her the practitioner is also helping to preserve and protect the patient's autonomy,"[8] a view that is also endorsed by Chris Hackler.[9]

If this control-based account of privacy is correct, then it is a simple matter to show that violations of a person's privacy will also compromise her autonomy. On this account of privacy, when a person's privacy is violated, she loses control over certain aspects of information about herself or her affairs.[10] Since this is so, then through this violation of her privacy, a person will lose the ability to exercise her autonomy over whether or not she will divulge the information in question.

Yet this simple way of accounting for the purported relationship between privacy and autonomy rests upon a mischaracterization of the concept of privacy. As Judith Jarvis Thomson has noted, to define privacy as the possession of control over information is mistaken. To illustrate this, Thomson offers a counterexample to any attempt to define privacy in terms of control:

> If my neighbor invents an X-ray device which enables him to look through walls, then I should imagine I thereby lose control over who can look at me: going home and closing the doors no longer suffices to prevent others from doing so. But my . . . privacy is not violated until my neighbor actually does train the device on the wall of my house. It is the actual looking that violates it, not the acquisition of the power to look.[11]

Thomson is correct here. Even though a person might be unable to control whether or not anyone looks at her, her privacy has not been violated unless someone actually *does* look at her. The potential for the violation of one's privacy is simply that—a *potential* for the violation of one's privacy, not a violation of one's privacy itself. Furthermore, to provide additional support to Thomson's criticism here, one could also construct cases where a person *retains* control over who looks at her and yet *still* suffers a loss of privacy. Consider, for example, a person who is rather absentminded and frequently forgets to close her curtains while she undresses, so enabling her prurient neighbor to stand outside her bedroom and watch her. If he does so look he violates his neighbor's privacy, but she still retains control over whether or not he is able to see her; she can simply draw her curtains. Clearly, then, if privacy is not to be defined in terms of control, then the arguments that rely on this conception of privacy to demonstrate that a violation of one's privacy necessarily serves also to compromise one's autonomy will fail.

## THE PURPORTED NECESSARY CONNECTION BETWEEN PRIVACY AND AUTONOMY

Before considering additional arguments as to why violations of a person's privacy would necessarily compromise her autonomy it would be sensible to offer a working definition of privacy. It is plausible to hold that something is private if a person may justifiably refuse to allow it to be accessible to others without her consent. Thus, a person's property is private if she can justifiably refuse to allow others access to it, while her medical records would be private with respect to those persons that she can justifiably withhold them from. On this account, privacy is an inherently normative concept.[12] Moreover, it is also a relational concept. While a person might be justified in excluding some persons from a certain item of information, she might not be justified in excluding others from having access to the same information. For example, while a person might be justified in refusing to give her friends access to information about any hereditary genetic diseases she might be a carrier for, she would not be justified in refusing to give her spouse this information when they plan to have children. With these remarks in place, for the purposes of this chapter, something is private with respect to another entity (be this another person, a corporation, or the State) if its current possessor is justified in attempting to prevent that entity from gaining access to it.[13]

With this working account of privacy in place, one may now turn to further (and more persuasive) arguments that attempt to demonstrate that if a person's privacy is violated, then her autonomy will necessarily be compromised.[14] These arguments attempt to show that violations of privacy compromise personal autonomy in two main ways: Such violations inhibit the ability of an agent to develop her autonomy, or they inhibit her ability to exercise it once it has been developed, or both.

Joseph Kupfer focuses upon the first of these ways in which a diminution in the degree of privacy a person enjoys serves to compromise her autonomy, arguing, "privacy is essential to the development and maintenance of an autonomous self."[15] Kupfer's arguments are based upon a conception of privacy that "includes some control over some information about oneself" and a notion of autonomy that "necessarily includes a concept of oneself as a purposeful, self-determining, responsible agent."[16] With these working definitions of the core concepts in place, Kupfer argues that there are two ways in which a violation of an agent's privacy may inhibit her ability to develop into an autonomous person.

Kupfer argues that "privacy contributes to the formation and development of autonomous individuals by providing them with control over whether or not their psychological existence becomes part of another's experience. Just this sort of control is necessary for them to think of themselves as self-determining."[17] In support of this claim Kupfer cites Jean Piaget and Victor Tausk, whose work in child psychology appears to show that a child's growing sense of self is correlated to her understanding that she is able to control information about herself.[18] Thus, as the child begins to recognize that she is able to determine "whether and to what degree others have access to her . . . [she] develops an autonomous self-concept."[19] According to Kupfer, the possession of privacy is thus a necessary condition for one to develop the concept of oneself as a purposeful, self-determining, responsible agent that is required for one to become an autonomous person. There is thus a necessary connection between privacy and autonomy in that the possession of the former is required for the development of the latter.

Kupfer also argues that if a person does not enjoy privacy she will be unable fully to engage in self-reflection and self-criticism. Engaging in such self-reflection, Kupfer argues, enables a person to achieve a greater degree of self-knowledge, the possession of which would help her to develop and maintain her autonomy in two ways. Most simply, a person who is able to come to know herself better through such a private process of introspection is more likely to know her own weaknesses and, so will be in a better position to avoid situations where she may suffer from a loss of autonomy through their exploitation. In addition to this, Kupfer argues that the ability to "try things out" in private will also enable a person to critically reflect on her "deepest convictions about what a noble or good life consists in," free from the distracting (and heteronomy-inducing) intrusion of others.[20] Stanley I. Benn also offers an argument that is similar to this.[21] Benn argues that the enjoyment of privacy is necessary for a person to develop her autonomy, for if a person does not enjoy some measure of privacy, her actions will be subject to the critical scrutiny of others. Recognizing this, a person will alter her actions so as to avoid public disapprobation, or else simply to avoid looking foolish. To the degree that a person lacks privacy, then, Benn argues, her actions are more likely to be subject to the guiding force of public opinion—a situation that would foster heteronomy rather than autonomy.[22] Thus, argue both Benn and Kupfer, the violation of a person's privacy will necessarily compromise her autonomy through inhibiting her development of a self-concept that is sufficiently robust to ground her possession of the capacity for autonomous thought and action.

## AUTONOMY AND PRIVACY REVISITED

Both Kupfer and Benn fail to demonstrate the truth of their claims that if one's privacy is violated, one's autonomy will thereby be compromised because they both fail to distinguish between overt and covert violations of privacy.

An overt violation of privacy is one in which the person whose privacy is being violated is aware of this fact. The most obvious example of such an overt violation of privacy is the violation of Winston Smith's privacy by the omnipresent surveillance of Big Brother in George Orwell's *1984*. By contrast, a covert violation of privacy is one in which the victim is unaware that she is under observation. Being watched by a well-hidden Peeping Tom or having one's room bugged in the Watergate Hotel are both ways in which a person's privacy might be covertly violated. Once this distinction between overt and covert violations of privacy has been made explicit, it is immediately striking that the arguments of both Kupfer and Benn focused solely upon the autonomy-compromising nature of overt violations of privacy. This is important, for one could covertly violate the privacy of another (i.e., observe her without her knowledge or suspicion) without thereby compromising her autonomy in any of the ways they outline.

To see this, let us turn to Kupfer's first example. If a child merely *believed* that she was able to control who was able to sense her, this would suffice to engender within her the belief "that many things remain hidden unless she chooses to reveal them," a belief that will in turn lead her to believe that she has "some power to determine what happens to her." The child, then, need not possess any *actual* privacy to develop the conception of herself as an agent who is able to control aspects of her environment that Kupfer argues is necessary for her to possess if she is to develop into an autonomous agent. Instead, she need only have the belief that she is able to control who may "sense" her to develop this self-concept—and the development and maintenance of this belief is quite compatible with her being continuously subjected to covert surveillance. Similarly, a person need not possess any actual privacy to engage in the sort of self-reflection that Kupfer believes is important to the development and maintenance of an autonomous self. Rather, all a person needs in order for her to engage in such autonomy-enhancing activities is the belief that she is performing them in private. This point can also be made with respect to Benn's claims concerning the relationship between privacy and autonomy. Instead of needing to enjoy genuine privacy in order to avoid heteronomously succumbing to the pressures of popular opinion, all a person needs to feel free to practice her independent judgment is the belief that she is doing so in private. Once again, then, a person need not actually enjoy privacy in order to participate in (and benefit from) the autonomy-developing and autonomy-enhancing activities that Benn and Kupfer focus on.

## THE PROBLEM OF COVERT SURVEILLANCE

Through failing to distinguish between overt and covert violations of privacy, the closest connection between personal autonomy and privacy that Kupfer establishes is that it is necessary for a child not to be subjected to overt violations of her privacy if she is to develop into an autonomous agent. But this is not the same as the claim that a person's currently existing capacity for autonomy will be compromised through a violation of her privacy. Moreover, Kupfer and Benn also only establish that there is a contingent connection between a person having her privacy *overtly* violated and her suffering from compromised autonomy. This connection is contingent because a person who was indifferent to the views of others would not be deterred from publicly living as she wished by the worry that she might be subjected to ridicule. Such a person would thus not require privacy to be immune from the heteronomy-inducing effects of public opinion. Thus, the arguments of Kupfer and Benn both depend here on the assumption that the person in question is motivated to modify her behavior in light of public opinion.

To develop a connection between violations of a person's privacy *per se* and the compromising of her autonomy, then, one must focus not just on the effects that overt violations of privacy have on their victim's autonomy but also on the effects that covert violations of her privacy have as well.

At first sight, the claim that covert violations of privacy can compromise the autonomy of persons appears implausible. To see this, consider a simple thought experiment. In World One, Jim is free from covert surveillance and directs his life in accordance with his own values and desires, enjoying a high degree of autonomy as he does so. In World Two, however, Twin Jim is (quite unsuspectingly) constantly subject to covert surveillance; his privacy is continuously violated. However, since he suspects nothing of this, he lives his life exactly as does Jim of World One, directing his actions in accordance with his own values and desires. Since the lives of Jim and Twin Jim are (apparently) identical with respect to the decisions that they make, the desires that they have, and the actions that they perform, it is unclear why one should claim that Twin Jim's autonomy is compromised and Jim's is not. And yet this is precisely the claim that must be supported if one is to accept the standard view that a violation of one's privacy will also compromise one's autonomy.

Although this thought experiment casts doubt upon the plausibility of the standard claim concerning the relationship between privacy and autonomy, there is a way in which it may be shown that Twin Jim's autonomy with respect to his decisions and actions *is* compromised in a way that Jim's is not. Despite first appearances, the decisions and actions of a person who is subject to covert surveillance might be subject to the *control* of a third party. A person who covertly violates the privacy of another might be able to exercise control over a subset of her beliefs (namely, whether or not she is being observed), and, through this, exercise control over her decisions and actions. Thus, insofar as a person suffers from the compromise of her autonomy if someone else controls what decisions she makes and hence what actions she performs, the victim of covert surveillance whose decisions and actions are subject to the control of another in this way might thereby suffer from compromised autonomy with respect to them.

## PRIVACY, BELIEF CONTROL, AND AUTONOMY

A straightforward analysis of how a covert violator of privacy can control the desires and actions of his victim through controlling her beliefs can be drawn from Daniel C. Dennett's analysis of control. Here, "A controls B if and only if the relation between A and B is such that A can drive B into whichever of B's normal range of states A wants B to be in."[23] A person who places another under covert surveillance will be able to exert such control over whether or not his victim believes that she is being watched. If he wishes her to believe that she is being watched, and so act accordingly, he can simply reveal himself. Alternatively, he can remain hidden, and allow her to continue to act on the false belief that she is enjoying a measure of privacy. It is thus up to the surveiller what type of actions his surveillee will decide to perform; those that she deems suitable for public view, or those she deems suitable only for private performance. Since it is thus he who is deciding what type of actions she will desire to perform, and not she, she will involuntarily suffer from a diminution in her autonomy with respect to the decisions that she makes and the actions that she performs while under covert surveillance.

Although this use of Dennett's account of control appears to explain how a covert surveiller may control the decisions, and hence actions, of his victim and so compromise her autonomy, as it stands this account of control is subject to counterexamples and so cannot be used for this purpose. To see this, consider the case of an exceptionally Plausible Liar, who knows that he will be able to convince his Gullible Friend of anything that he wishes. Since this is so, the Plausible Liar knows that he may drive his friend into making any decisions that he wishes her to make simply by instilling in her the appropriate beliefs that (either alone or in conjunction with her preexisting desires) would lead her to make them. When the Plausible Liar lies to his Gullible Friend to get her to make a certain decision he will, on Dennett's analysis of control, be in control of her decisions, and so she will suffer from a diminution in her autonomy with respect to them. This is certainly a correct conclusion to draw—and one that is fully supported by the analysis of autonomy that was developed in Chapter 1. However, on Dennett's analysis of control the Plausible Liar *does not actually have to lie* to control the decisions of his Gullible Friend. For Dennett, "A controls B if and only if . . . A *can* drive B into whichever of B's normal range of states A wants B to be in" (emphasis added). Since the Plausible Liar *can* drive his Gullible Friend into making the decisions that he wishes her to make, he satisfies this condition for controlling her *even if* he does not actually lie to her. Since this is so, on Dennett's view, the Plausible Liar's friend will be under his control (and thus will suffer from a diminution in her autonomy) *whenever* he is in a position to lie to her, even if he sticks strictly to the truth. And this will be the case even if the Plausible Liar *does not realize* that he has this ability and so never attempts to exercise it. Whether he realizes it or not, the Plausible Liar *can* direct the decisions of his Gullible Friend in this way—and this ability is all that is needed on Dennett's analysis for him to be in control of her. However, it is not the case that simply because the Plausible Liar *can* control his Gullible Friend that he *is* exerting control over her. To reprise Thomson's objection to the characterization of privacy as control, just because the Plausible Liar has the *potential* to control his friend's desires does not mean that he is *actually* exercising such control. Therefore, Dennett's analysis of control should not be accepted as it stands—and so neither should the prior account of a covert violation of a person's privacy serve to compromise her autonomy.

It should be noted that Dennett's account of control is subject to this Thomson-style objection because (as it is written) its antecedent clause is described in terms of what is actually the case, whereas its consequent clause is described in counterfactual terms. Dennett is committed to claiming that A controls B if A can drive B into any one of B's normal range of states, even if A does not actually do so. And this claim is mistaken: That A has the *ability* to drive B into any of B's normal range of states is not the same as A's *exercise* of this ability. To avoid this difficulty, Dennett's analysis of control should be revised to read that "A controls B if and only if the relation between A and B is such that A actually drives B into whichever of B's normal range of states A wants B to be in."

Before using this revised Dennettian account of control to provide an analysis of how a person's being subject to covert surveillance might compromise her autonomy, one should recall the outline of the model of human motivation that this analysis will be based upon, and that has been both implicitly (in Chapters 2 and 3) and explicitly (in the previous chapter) undergirding the account of practical autonomy that has been the mainstay of this volume. On this model of human motivation persons possess a set of core desires that underlie many of their motivations.[24] Some of these core desires will be hardwired biological needs (such as the need for food and the need for pleasure) that will be shared by all persons. Others will be peculiar to a particular person, what Bernard Williams terms a person's "commitments," the particular attachments that give meaning and purpose to her life. These core desires will not usually specify their objects in precise terms.[25] Instead, a person will form a first-order desire with a specific intentional object as a result of these core desires combining with her beliefs about what will satisfy them.

With this model in hand, it is clear that A can exert Dennettian control over the decisions that B makes (and hence over the subsequent first-order desires that she has, and the actions that she performs) to the degree that he is able to control her beliefs. If A controls B's beliefs, he will be able to use this control to channel the intentionality of her core motivations so that B makes the decisions that he wants her to make, and her effective first-order desires have the objects that he wishes. Moreover, A can achieve this either through causing B to possess certain beliefs through lying to her or deceiving her or through ensuring that B continues to have the beliefs that she has (and that he wishes her to continue to possess) by withholding information from her that would cause her to alter her doxastic state.

Once this Dennettian account of control has been combined with this account of human motivation, one can explain how even a covert violation of a person's privacy might compromise her autonomy. As was noted previously in the original attempt to offer such a control-based explanation when one person places another under covert surveillance, he acts so as to prevent her from discovering that she is being watched. He thus acts so as to control what beliefs she has concerning whether or not she is being watched. If he is successful in exercising this control, he will thus control the type of actions that she decides to perform: those that she deems suitable for public view or those she considers to be the type that she would only perform in private. Since (from Chapter 1) a person enjoys autonomy with respect to her decisions and her consequent actions to the extent that she, and not someone else, controls her performance of them, when a surveiller usurps control over his surveillee's decisions and actions in this way he compromises her autonomy with respect to them. Covert violations of a person's privacy, then, might indeed serve to compromise her autonomy.[26]

## REFINING THIS ACCOUNT

Arguing that a covert violation of a person's privacy *might* also serve to compromise her autonomy is not, of course, to argue in favor of the received view in the literature on privacy and autonomy; namely, that a violation of a person's privacy *necessarily* results in the compromise of her autonomy. As such, then, it does not support the view, common in bioethics, that concern for patient confidentiality is based on concern for the value of patient autonomy on the grounds that a violation of the former will lead to a compromise of the latter. Rather, to argue in this way is only to accept that there is a *contingent* relationship between a person's possession of privacy and her enjoyment of autonomy. To provide a full account of the relationship between the possession of privacy and the enjoyment of autonomy, then, one must outline the various additional conditions that must be met if a covert violation of a person's privacy is also to compromise her autonomy.

The first of these conditions focuses on the conative state of the person who is subject to covert surveillance. In the prior discussion it was implicitly assumed that the person subject to covert surveillance would decide to alter her behavior once she realized that she was being watched. If, however, the surveillee did not care whether or not she was being watched, she would not decide to alter the type of actions that she performs were she to come to discover that she was under covert surveillance. If this were so, then the surveiller would be unable to affect what decisions his surveillee made through either revealing himself or continuing covertly to observe. This is because the beliefs of the surveillee that are under the surveiller's control (i.e., those that concern whether her actions are observed or unobserved) would not be those that would play a role in her decisions concerning which actions to perform. This being so, for a person to suffer from compromised autonomy when she is subjected to covert violations of her privacy she must be disposed to alter her behavior if she believes that she is under observation.

The second condition that must be met for a covert violation of a person's privacy to compromise her autonomy is similar to the first. Just as a person whose decisions would be unaffected by the knowledge that she was under observation is immune to having her autonomy compromised through covert violations of her privacy, so too is a person whose decisions would be affected by such knowledge but who already believes that she is under such surveillance.[27] Such a person would already have decided to perform the type of actions that she considered it would be appropriate for her to perform while being observed. This being so, the control that the covert surveiller would otherwise have been able to exercise over this person's beliefs is lost, for it is now no longer up to him whether or not she believes that she is being observed. Thus, for a person to be vulnerable to having her autonomy compromised through covert violations of her privacy, she must both have the desire to alter her actions if she discovers that she is under observation and also lack the belief that she is under observation.

The third and fourth conditions that must be met in order for a covert violation of a person's privacy also to compromise her autonomy focus on the abilities and mental states of the surveiller, rather than the surveillee. The third condition follows from the first two: that for a person's autonomy to be compromised through a covert violation of her privacy the person who violates her privacy must be able to exercise control over those of the surveillee's beliefs that are relevant to her decision-making procedures. If a covert surveiller is unable to let the person whose privacy he is covertly violating know that her privacy is being violated, he will be unable to affect her beliefs in the way that is required for him to exercise control over what decisions she makes and what actions she performs, and his covert observation of such a person will not compromise her autonomy. For example, when Scrooge visited his nephew in the company of the Ghost of Christmas Past in *A Christmas Carol*, he was unable to inform his relatives of his presence as he watched their domestic Christmas activities. Thus, even though Scrooge was covertly violating the privacy of his nephew and his family, he was not thereby compromising their autonomy. Owing to his inability to alert them to his presence, he was unable to exercise any control over whether or not they believed they were observed, and, since he thus could not control their beliefs, he could not control either their decisions or their consequent actions. For a covert violation of a person's privacy also to compromise her autonomy, then, the person who is violating her privacy must be able to communicate to her that she is being observed.

The final condition focuses on the mental states of the covert violator of privacy. This condition is owed to the recognition (argued for in Chapter 1, through the examples of Iago and Othello, and McIago and McOthello) that for one person to compromise the autonomy of another through subjecting her to control, it must be the case that the controller intends to exercise such control over the controllee. Given this, it is a necessary (but not a sufficient) condition for person A to control person B in such that B's autonomy with respect to her consequent decisions and actions is compromised that *A* must *intend* to control B. Since this is so, for a person's autonomy to be compromised through her being subject to a covert violation of her privacy, the violator of her privacy must *intend* to exert control over the decisions that she makes and the type of actions that she performs. Thus, the final condition that must be met for a covert violation of a person's privacy to compromise her autonomy is that the covert violator of her privacy must intend to control whether his surveillee performed those actions that she believed were suitable for public consumption or those she believed should only be performed in private.

This last condition enables one to provide an intuitively plausible account of cases in which a person's privacy is covertly yet inadvertently violated. One example of such an inadvertent covert violation of privacy would be where a person is walking along a street after dark and happens to glance up at a lighted window where he sees a couple embracing. In this case, it would be odd to claim that the couple suffered from a diminution in their autonomy with respect to the decisions that they made for the brief moment in which they were observed, with their autonomy being fully restored to them as soon as the inadvertent (and no doubt embarrassed) Peeping Tom looked away. Given the fourth condition, however, one need not claim that the couple's autonomy was compromised in this way. They were subject to an *inadvertent* violation of their privacy.[28] Since the inadvertent Peeping Tom did not intend to exert control over the desires and actions of this couple by deliberately violating their privacy, the final condition that is required for a covert violator of privacy also thereby to compromise the autonomy of those he covertly observes is not met. Thus, the autonomy of this couple was not compromised, for the violator of their privacy did not intend to exert control over what type of desires they possessed and actions they performed.

## AUTONOMY AND OVERT VIOLATIONS OF PRIVACY

It is now clear that the widely accepted claim that a violation of a person's privacy will necessarily compromise her autonomy is false, for there is only a contingent connection between the covert violation of a person's privacy and the compromise of her autonomy—a connection that is dependent upon the four other conditions outlined previously being met in addition to that of the covert violation of a person's privacy. Moreover, from the prior discussion of how a covert violation of a person's privacy might compromise her autonomy, it has become clear how a comprehensive analysis of the relationship between privacy and autonomy should be developed. This discussion has shown that to determine whether a given violation of privacy (either overt or covert) also compromises the autonomy of the person so affected, one needs to ascertain whether this violation enabled the violator to usurp control over the decisions that this person made and hence the actions that she was motivated to perform.

Just as a covert violator of a person's privacy might compromise her autonomy through usurping control over her belief as to whether or not she is being watched, so too might an *overt* violator of a person's privacy compromise her autonomy through affecting her beliefs in the same way. When a person *believes* that she is subject to an overt violation of privacy, she will adjust her behavior so that she only performs actions that she is willing to be observed performing. (As was discussed previously, for this to be true the person concerned must care about what actions she is observed performing.) As Kupfer, Benn, and Rachels argue, then, a person who is subject to overt violations of her privacy, and who realizes this, might modify her behavior to avoid the disapprobation (or to secure the approbation) of those she believes are watching her. (Similarly, a person who is deliberately fooled into believing that she is being observed when she is not, and who adjusts her behavior accordingly, will also suffer from a diminution in her autonomy with respect to her decisions and her consequent actions.) A person whose privacy is overtly violated (and who cares about the opinions of her surveillers) will thus be effectively acting under duress; she will act in the way that she believes will please her observers, who will otherwise impose upon her the penalties of ridicule or disapprobation. The actions that such a person will perform to avoid such disapprobation will thus not exemplify her own values (except insofar as she values avoiding the disapprobation or ridicule of her observers) but what she believes the values of her observers to be. To the extent that this is so, then, such a person will not be fully autonomous with respect to them.[29]

## AUTONOMY AND PATIENT CONFIDENTIALITY

From the previous discussion it is clear that the widely accepted claim that a violation of a person's privacy will also compromise her autonomy is false. This, however, should not lead one to claim that there is no connection between violations of a person's privacy and the compromising of her autonomy—and so it should not lead one immediately to reject the view that concern for patient confidentiality is based on concern for patient autonomy. Instead, it should be recognized that insofar as there is a *contingent* connection between violations of a person's privacy and the compromise of her autonomy certain violations of a person's medical confidentiality could indeed serve to compromise her autonomy. As such, then, given the value of autonomy in contemporary bioethics one should err on the side of caution and adopt a default position that out of respect for patient autonomy one should respect patient confidentiality, for if one does not do so there is a possibility that one's violation of a patient's privacy could lead to the compromise of her autonomy.

Yet despite the plausibility of this as a default position—and despite its appeal as a nonrevisionary approach to the practical effects of the theoretical discussion of the relationship between patient privacy and patient autonomy—the discussion of the relationship between privacy and autonomy in this chapter should lead one to feel disquieted about this conclusion. In recognizing that the relationship between violating a person's privacy and compromising her autonomy was merely a contingent one it was recognized that for the violation of a person's privacy also to compromise her autonomy four further conditions must be met: (i) the person whose privacy was violated must care about such a violation, such that she would make decisions in a situation in which she believed that she was being watched that would be different from those she would make were she not to have this belief; (ii) the person whose privacy is violated does not currently believe that her privacy is being violated; (iii) the violator of her privacy can control whether or not he informs her that he is violating her privacy; and (iv) the violator of her privacy violates it with the intention of exerting some degree of control over which decisions she makes. It is clear that conditions (i) to (iii) will frequently be met when a person's medical confidentiality is breached. It is also clear, however, that condition (iv) will frequently *not* be met. A healthcare professional might, for example, provide information about her patients' medical conditions to persons engaged in epidemiological research, including as she does so information (such as address and date of birth) that is not only relevant to the research in question, but which would enable the researchers to identify the patients whose medical information they had access to should they desire to do so.[30] Such a provision of information would clearly breach the privacy of the patients whose information was supplied to the researchers—yet, since it was not done with the intent of exerting control over their decisions or actions it would not serve to compromise their autonomy. As such, then, it would seem that a moral concern for patient autonomy could not serve as a justification for moral strictures against such breaches of patient confidentiality. Thus, insofar as such breaches are morally condemned, the reason for such condemnation must be based on something other than a concern for patient autonomy.

This argument, however, moves too fast. Although it is plausible to hold that certain breaches of patient privacy will not compromise the autonomy of those subject to them this does not show that respect for the value of patient autonomy is not the underlying concern that justifies a concern with maintaining patient confidentiality. To see this it should be recognized that one reason why persons are concerned about breaches of patient confidentiality even if these do not compromise the autonomy of those subject to them is that such breaches would foster patient mistrust of healthcare providers. If there is not a strong ethical proscription in favor of maintaining patient confidentiality persons are likely to be less willing to disclose information to their healthcare providers that is pertinent to their condition, or even to avoid healthcare providers altogether when they believe that they have conditions that they do not wish others to know of (e.g., socially stigmatized diseases or conditions that could adversely affect their actuarial status). Such mistrust of the healthcare profession would be likely to result in persons being able to use their autonomy less effectively than they would be able to in its absence, for it would discourage them from using it to secure their health-related goals. As such, then, even if breaches of patient confidentiality would not themselves compromise the autonomy of those patients subject to them, concern for the *instrumental* value of patient autonomy could still indirectly undergird concern for patient privacy.

## CONCLUSION

In this chapter it was argued that the widespread belief that a violation of a person's privacy would necessarily serve to compromise her autonomy is mistaken. Instead, there is merely a contingent connection between the violation of a person's privacy and the compromise of her autonomy. Moreover—and of concern to persons interested in bioethics—that connection is one that would not be present in many cases in which a person's privacy with respect to her medical records is violated. That this is so does not, however, show that a concern for the value of patient autonomy does not undergird the ethical concern with maintaining patient confidentiality, for the maintenance of such confidentiality can be justified indirectly, through appeal to the instrumental value of patient (or potential patient) autonomy. This conclusion might appear simply to support the generally accepted view that concern for patient autonomy is the ethical foundation of concern for patient confidentiality, and so to be less than theoretically exciting. But although this is true in part insofar as it is concern for the instrumental value of patient autonomy that provides this ethical foundation, it is now clear that the relationship between respect for autonomy and respect for patient confidentiality is not as direct as it is often believed. With this point in hand, the next chapter will consider another area in which a concern for personal autonomy is supposed to support another generally accepted bioethical requirement: the need to secure a patient's informed consent to her treatment.

# 9  Autonomy and Informed Consent

## INTRODUCTION

The view that concern for autonomy provides the ethical foundation for the doctrine of informed consent has come to be accepted as a truism within contemporary medical ethics. In their seminal work, *Principles of Biomedical Ethics*, for example, Beauchamp and Childress maintain that the "the primary justification advanced for requirements of informed consent has been to protect autonomous choice."[1] Similarly, Faden and Beauchamp claim that an "analysis of the nature of autonomy provides the essential foundation for our analysis of the nature of informed consent," while Appelbaum, Lidz, and Meisel hold that informed consent is "an ethical doctrine, rooted in our society's cherished value of autonomy."[2] Moreover, the view that concern for autonomy provides the foundation for informed consent is not peculiar to bioethics; it is also received wisdom in legal discussions of this doctrine. For example, in the case that started the serious legal discussion of informed consent, *Canterbury v. Spence*, it was insisted that informed consent is required to secure "the patient's right of self-determination."[3]

Yet, just as in the previous chapter it was noted that very few arguments have been advanced to support the conventional view that concern for patient autonomy is the ethical foundation of concern for patient privacy, so too have few sustained arguments been offered for the conventional view that the ethical foundation of informed consent is concern for autonomy. And just as this paucity of argument was regrettable in the context of discussions of patient confidentiality, for, as was argued in the previous chapter, the connection between a violation of a person's privacy and the compromising of her autonomy is not as straightforward as it might at first appear, so too is it regrettable in the context of discussions of informed consent, for there appears to be good reason to believe that concern for autonomy is not the ethical basis for informed consent. This is because in the context of seeking medical advice from a healthcare provider a person will only suffer from a diminution in her autonomy with respect to her medical decisions if she is manipulated or deceived by her healthcare provider, and she then unwittingly makes the decisions that her healthcare provider intended her to make as a result of his manipulation or deception.[4] As such, then, if a patient simply lacks information that is relevant to her medical decisions, and this lack is not owed to the deliberate acts or omissions of her health-care provider, she can be fully autonomous with respect to her medical decisions.[5] Her autonomy with respect to her medical decisions would thus not be compromised if her healthcare provider fails to secure her informed consent to her treatment as a result of negligently (i.e., unintentionally) omitting to provide relevant information to her. If the ethical foundation of the doctrine of informed consent is really concern for autonomy, then, it seems that such a negligent healthcare provider would not be morally culpable for his negligence, for such negligence would not have compromised his patient's autonomy. However, since it is counterintuitive to hold that healthcare providers are not morally culpable for negligently failing to secure their patients' informed consent to their treatment then it seems cannot be the case that the ethical foundation of the doctrine of informed consent is concern for autonomy.

This argument against the conventional view that concern for autonomy is the ethical foundation of informed consent will be developed further next, and defended against objections that have been leveled against it by Jukka Varelius. With this argument and defense in hand, it will then be argued that, as with the claim that concern for autonomy is the ethical foundation of concern for patient confidentiality, the view that concern for autonomy is the ethical foundation of informed consent can be defended by focusing on the instrumental value of autonomy.

## THE CONVENTIONAL VIEW OF AUTONOMY AND INFORMED CONSENT

It is not difficult to see why it is believed that concern for autonomy is the ethical foundation of the doctrine of informed consent. As Thomas May notes, "Autonomy involves steering the direction of one's life, determining how to behave, and deciding what projects to engage in"—a view of autonomy that has been more precisely captured in the account of practical autonomy that was developed in Chapter 1.[6] In order for a patient to be autonomous with respect to her decision to undergo certain medical treatments, then, her healthcare provider should not control her decision. He should not, for example, fail to disclose the possibility of a certain course of treatment to her that he believes would be inappropriate for her to pursue to prevent her from doing so, nor should he misrepresent her options to her for the same purpose.[7] If he does control her decisions through selectively presenting information about her medical options to her, it would be he, and not she, who was steering the direction of that part of her life, and so her autonomy with respect to those decisions concerning her medical treatment that he had affected would be compromised. To avoid healthcare professionals usurping the autonomy of their patients in this way, then, they should provide them with unbiased information about the alternative courses of treatment that are available to them and their respective advantages and disadvantages. The requirement that a patient give her informed consent to her treatment, then, appears to be based firmly on concern for her autonomy.

## NEGLIGENCE, INFORMED CONSENT, AND PATIENT AUTONOMY

The temptation to argue from the claim that informed consent precludes a person's healthcare provider from compromising her autonomy through usurping control over her medical decisions to the claim that the ethical foundation for informed consent is concern for patient autonomy should, however, be resisted.[8] This is because it is possible for a person to fail to give her informed consent to a procedure and yet not suffer from any diminution in her autonomy with respect to her treatment decisions. In such cases where patient autonomy is not compromised, the healthcare provider would still be held to be morally culpable for failing to secure his patient's informed consent. Since this is so, concern for autonomy *per se* cannot be the ethical foundation for this doctrine. If it were, no blame should attach to the healthcare provider whose failure to secure his patient's informed consent did not adversely affect her autonomy.

To show that a person can fail to give his informed consent to a certain course of treatment and yet still be fully autonomous with respect to his decision to pursue it, it should be recalled that, as was argued for in Chapter 1 through the example of Iago and Othello, and McIago and McOthello, and noted again in the previous chapter, for one person to exert control over the decisions and actions of another in such a way that the first person acts to compromise the autonomy of the second, the first person must *intend* to exert control over the second. A patient's autonomy with respect to her treatment decisions would be compromised if her healthcare provider withheld information about her treatment options from her, or misrepresented them to her, to control her treatment decisions. This is because if a person's healthcare provider controls the information that is available to her he will be able to control her beliefs about her options, and so will be able to control the decisions that she makes on the basis of those beliefs. Furthermore, to the extent that a patient's healthcare provider has knowledge of her desires and values, he will be able to control what decisions the patient makes by, Iago-like, adjusting the information that she receives about her treatment options to ensure that she makes the medical decisions that he desires her to make. Thus, if a healthcare provider exercises such control over his patient's decisions, then it will be he, and not she, who directs her decisions, and to the extent that this is so the patient will not be autonomous with respect to them.

It is important to recall here that for one person to exercise control over the decisions of a patient in this way he must intentionally filter the information that she receives to direct her to make the decisions that he wants her to make. Thus, were a third person to provide a patient with the same information as did her controlling healthcare provider, and yet not do so in order to exert control over her decisions, he would not usurp control over her decisions, and so her autonomy with respect to them would be unimpaired.

If it is a necessary condition for A to exert control over the decisions of B in that A must intend to do this then if a healthcare provider negligently (i.e., unintentionally) omits to provide relevant information to a patient concerning her treatment, he would not thereby be exerting control over her. Thus, if a healthcare provider negligently omits to secure his patient's informed consent to her treatment he will not thereby have compromised her autonomy with respect to her treatment decisions, for he would not be acting with the intent to control them. In illustration of this, consider the case of *Cobbs v. Grant*. In this case the Supreme Court of California found that Grant had been negligent in failing to disclose to Cobbs that one of the risks of surgery performed to relieve a duodenal ulcer is that a new ulcer might develop.[9] Grant did not fail to disclose this risk to Cobbs because he intended to influence Cobbs's decision concerning the treatment of his ulcer. Instead, as he argued in court, he had merely followed common medical practice in which risks that had a low probability of transpiring were not disclosed to the patient. Grant thus did not exert control over Cobbs, because even though he failed to disclose to Cobbs one of the risks of his surgery, this failure to disclose did not result from Grant's intending to thus exert control over Cobbs. Instead, Grant simply presented all the information that he believed he should present to Cobbs to him and allowed him to make his own decisions in the light of it. Cobbs was thus not under the control of Grant. He directed himself to undergo the surgery for his ulcer and was fully autonomous with respect to this decision.

Yet even though Cobbs was autonomous with respect to his decision to undergo surgery for his ulcer, he did not give his informed consent to this operation, for he was unaware of the risks that were associated with it. A person, then, can fail to give his informed consent to a medical procedure and yet not suffer from any diminution in his autonomy with respect to his decision to undergo it. If concern for patient autonomy is the ethical foundation for requiring that a person give his informed consent to his medical treatment, then healthcare providers who negligently fail to secure informed consent from their patients would not be morally culpable for this, because this failure would not result in their patients' autonomy being compromised. But to hold that a healthcare provider who negligently fails to secure a patient's informed consent is not morally culpable for such failure is highly counterintuitive. Since this is so, it appears that concern for autonomy is not the ethical foundation for the doctrine of informed consent.[10]

## AN OBJECTION TO THIS ARGUMENT
## AGAINST THE CONVENTIONAL VIEW

There are two initial objections to this argument against the conventional claim that concern for patient autonomy is the ethical foundation of the doctrine of informed consent. The first is based on the claim that a person's autonomy with respect to his decisions might be compromised if he did not understand their implications. Here, one might argue that the person concerned would be unable to direct his life to achieve his goals, since he would be ignorant of which actions he should take to achieve this; a person who did not understand the implications of his actions would fail to direct himself in accord with desires and values—he would not be autonomous with respect to any of his decisions that he made in ignorance. Applying this reasoning to the case of Othello, a proponent of this objection would claim that in both *Othello* and *McOthello* both Othello and McOthello suffered from compromised autonomy, because they acted in ignorance of their true situation. Thus, such a proponent would continue, Grant did compromise the autonomy of Cobbs through failing to disclose the effects of his surgery to him, because Cobbs's ignorance of the effects precluded him from successfully directing himself in accordance with his desires and values. Since even a negligent failure on the part of a healthcare provider to secure her patient's informed consent would thus on this view compromise his autonomy, the argument against the conventional view of the relationship between autonomy and informed consent fails.

The objection is based on the view that for a person to be autonomous with respect to his decisions and actions he must exhibit a certain degree of comprehension of what he is doing. (As Beauchamp and Childress put it, autonomy is incompatible with inadequate understanding that prevents meaningful choice.[11]) This objection is thus one that is internal to the account of practical autonomy developed in this volume. This is because (as was argued in Chapter 7 against the extreme voluntarist position), for a person's decisions to be ones that he was autonomous with respect to he must direct himself to make them, and such self-direction necessarily involves the person in question making his decisions on the basis of his own desires and values. For a person to be autonomous with respect to his decisions, then, he must have some understanding of what he is deciding to do, where this understanding is both descriptive (he has an understanding of what he is deciding to do) and normative (he places a certain value on what he intends his actions to being about). But to hold that a person must understand what he is doing to a degree that is sufficient for his decisions and choices to be meaningful ones is compatible with his being ignorant of the most salient intensional description of the actions that he is deciding to perform. Note that whether or not an intensional description of an action is the most salient one will be affected by whether one is concerned with assessing the prudence of performing the action in question or the praise or blame that should be attributed to its performer. If one is interested in assessing the prudence of a person's performing an action one will assess the degree to which its performance is likely to enable her to achieve the ends that she wishes to achieve through its performance.[12] If one is interested in assessing the praise or blame that should be attributed to the person who performed it one will be interested in assessing both the morality of the act in question and the presence or absence of any conditions that would mitigate her responsibility for it. To see that a person can be autonomous with respect to his decisions and actions even if they are made and performed in ignorance of their most salient intensional descriptions consider the examples of Martin Frobisher's expeditions to the New World discussed in Chapter 1, and (given certain religious assumptions) the crucifixion of Jesus. Frobisher, recall, mistakenly loaded up his ship with Canadian iron pyrites in the belief that he was loading it with gold. Despite his acting in ignorance of the most prudentially salient intensional description of his action, however, as was noted in Chapter 1, it is still both natural and correct to hold that he was autonomous with respect both to his decision to so load his ship and to his consequent actions, even though neither his decision nor his actions led to him achieving his goal of returning to Britain with a ship full of gold. He was autonomous with respect to both his decisions and his consequent actions simply because a person is autonomous with respect to his decisions and his actions if it is he, and not someone else, who directs his performance of them, whether or not they actually lead to the person concerned achieving his goals through them. Similarly, Jesus' executioners were certainly autonomous with respect to his execution, for, like Frobisher, it was they, and not someone else, who directed their decisions and actions that led them to execute Him, even if these decisions and actions were made and performed in ignorance of their most morally salient intensional descriptions—namely, that they were killing the Son of God.[13] Thus, even though Cobbs's ignorance of the risks associated with his surgery might have compromised his ability to direct himself in a way that would be most likely to lead to the satisfaction of his desires and achievement of his goals, he still directed himself with respect to his decisions and consequent actions, and so he was still autonomous with respect to both his decisions and the actions that they moved him to perform.[14] That a healthcare provider's negligence might result in her patient being ignorant of information that would affect his decisions concerning his medical treatment in a way that would adversely affect his ability to satisfy his desires or achieve his medical goals, thus does not show that this patient's autonomy was thereby also compromised.

## RESPECTING AUTONOMY AND COMPROMISING AUTONOMY

The second objection to the prior argument against the conventional view of the relationship between autonomy and informed consent is that it does not allow us to distinguish between *compromising* the autonomy of a person and *failing to respect it*. If a physician ignores her patient's desire not to be medicated for her depression and writes her a prescription for Prozac, her failure to engage with her patient's autonomous request evinces a failure on her part to respect his autonomy.[15] However, even though she might *fail to respect* her patient's autonomy, the physician does not thereby *compromise* it, since she does not usurp any control over his desires or actions. It is still the patient, and not his physician, who will decide whether or not he will fill the prescription and take the drug. Conversely, a physician might act to compromise her patient's autonomy *because* she respects it. For example, a physician whose grossly obese patient requests that she place him in a facility where he will be forced to diet and exercise could respect his autonomy by acceding to his request, although this would lead to his autonomy being compromised for the duration of his incarceration.[16] It may be urged, then, that that a healthcare provider's negligent failure to secure her patient's informed consent to his treatment does not compromise his autonomy is not sufficient to show that no affront to his autonomy has occurred. Through her negligence, the healthcare provider might have failed to *respect* the autonomy of her patient—and this failure to respect autonomy provides grounds for holding the negligent healthcare provider morally culpable, irrespective of whether or not her patient suffered from any *compromise* of his autonomy.

In response to this objection it should be noted that it is plausible to hold that for A to respect the autonomy of B she must intentionally allow him to make his own decisions in light of his own beliefs and values, and refrain from subjecting him to coercion, duress, manipulation, or deception. As such, it appears that a negligent healthcare provider would respect her patient's autonomy if she refrained from subjecting him to any of these autonomy-compromising influences. A healthcare provider's negligence would thus not preclude her from adopting a respectful attitude toward the autonomy of her patients and allowing them to make the decisions about their treatment that they see fit to make. It seems that even a negligent healthcare provider, then, cannot be held to be morally accountable for her negligence on the grounds that such negligence would evince a lack of respect for the autonomy of her patients. Thus, if negligent healthcare professionals are to be held to be morally culpable for their negligence, it seems that this cannot be because they act so as to compromise their patients' autonomy, or because they fail to respect it.

## RESPONSES TO VARELIUS

Jukka Varelius has argued that the previous argument that casts doubt on the view that concern for autonomy is the ethical foundation of informed consent is mistaken. Varelius holds that it rests on accepting four views, of which the three that are most immediately germane to this discussion are: (i) "that a person exerts control over the decisions and actions of another in such a way that the first person undermines the autonomy of the second only if the first person intends to exert control over the other"; (ii) "that maintaining that ignorance of relevant information undermines autonomy amounts to constructing autonomy as a success concept"; and (iii) "that a health care provider who negligently fails to secure his patient's informed consent to a treatment does not thereby fail to respect his patient's autonomy."[17] Varelius holds that none of these three views should be accepted, and so the argument that casts doubt on the conventional view of the relationship between autonomy and informed consent should be rejected.

Against the first of these views Varelius argues that "a person can suffer from a diminution in her autonomy with respect to her decisions and actions even if she is not intentionally controlled by others."[18] To support his view Varelius develops an example in which one person develops a drug with the intention of making another behave as he wants. He leaves the drug in the apartment of a third person, who takes the drug believing it to be aspirin. This third person then acts in accordance with the "irresistible desire to which the pills gave rise".[19] Although this third person's actions were "not the result of anyone else intentionally controlling her behavior . . . it would still be counterintuitive to claim that she was autonomous with respect to her doing what she did, since her doing what she did was caused by the drug that gives rise to an irresistible desire to do it."[20]

The response to this objection is simple. Varelius is correct to note that persons' autonomy could be compromised by the actions of others even if they did not intend them to have this effect. If, for example, I shoot mine arrow o'er the house and hurt my brother in such a way that I reduce him to the level of a contented infant I will certainly compromise his autonomy simpliciter through thereby eliminating his capacity for it, even though I did not intend this.[21] But that such unintentional compromisings of autonomy are possible does not show that the previous argument that casts doubt on the received view concerning the relationship between autonomy and informed consent is mistaken. This is because this argument does not rest on the view that a person can only suffer from a diminution in her autonomy with respect to her decisions and actions if she is intentionally controlled by another, as Varelius believes. Rather, it rests on the much more restricted view that when one person, A, provides (or refrains from providing) information to another, B, for A thereby to compromise the autonomy of B it is necessary that A provide (or refrain from providing) the information in question with the intention of thereby exerting control over B, such that B performs (or refrains from performing) the actions (or type of actions) that A desires her to perform (or to refrain from performing). Thus, since Varelius's purported counterexample does not address this more restricted view of the conditions that must be met for one person to act so as to compromise the autonomy of another (i.e., that which actually undergirds the previous argument against the conventional view of the relationship between autonomy and informed consent), it fails to show that the previous argument is not "acceptable."[22]

Varelius's objection to view (ii) is more successful, although it still fails to show that the previous argument should be rejected. In the original formulation of the previous argument against the conventional view of the relationship between autonomy and informed consent it was argued that to hold that a patient (e.g., Cobbs) must possess all existing information that he would need to make a decision concerning his medical treatment would be implausibly to construe autonomy as a success concept, such that a person would only be autonomous with respect to a decision that he made or an action that he performed if it actually led him to achieve the ends that he made it, or performed it, with the intention of achieving. Thus, it was held in the original formulation of this argument, since to construe autonomy as a success concept would be implausible, it must be the case that a person could be autonomous with respect to his decisions or his actions even if they were made, or performed, in ignorance of the relevant facts. As such, then, it was concluded, a patient could be fully autonomous with respect to his decisions and actions concerning his treatment even if his healthcare provider negligently failed to secure his informed consent to it.[23] As Varelius correctly notes, however, "If . . . we required that a person can make an autonomous medical decision concerning certain kinds of treatment only if she has all knowledge about her disease and the treatment in question that biomedical science has produced, this would not amount to constructing autonomy as a success concept," for "There simply is not enough knowledge concerning the disease and its treatment to guarantee success in achieving this person's goals."[24] However, although Varelius is correct to note that "requiring that an autonomous agent must have a certain amount of knowledge about the implications of her decisions and actions that can exceed the amount of information that some persons have without being informed by others need not result in constructing autonomy as a success concept" he provides no argument for the view that to be considered autonomous with respect to her decisions and actions an agent must have any particular degree of knowledge about the implications of her decisions and actions. As such, then, he has given no reason to believe that a person (such as Cobbs) who acted in ignorance of the most prudentially or morally salient intensional description of the actions that he decided to perform thereby suffered from a diminution in his autonomy with respect to the decisions and actions in question. This objection that Varelius has offered, then, does not undermine the previous argument against the conventional view of the relationship between autonomy and informed consent.[25]

With these responses to Varelius's objections to view (ii) in hand it is a simple matter to respond to his objection to (iii). Varelius objects to the view "that a health care provider who negligently fails to secure his patient's informed consent to a treatment does not thereby fail to respect his patient's autonomy" on the grounds that it is mistaken to believe that "decisions made in ignorance of relevant facts can be autonomous."[26] However, since Varelius's objections to (ii) are mistaken there is no reason to believe that his claim here is correct. As such, then, Varelius's objections to views (i) through (iii) inclusive can all be met.[27]

## INFORMED CONSENT AND THE INSTRUMENTAL VALUE OF PRACTICAL AUTONOMY

With these defenses of the above argument that casts doubt upon the conventional understanding of the relationship between autonomy and informed consent in hand it is now time to turn to a way in which it could be (partially) undermined. In response to the second initial objection to this argument it was held that all that is required for one person to respect the autonomy of another she must only refrain from subjecting him to coercion, duress, manipulation, or deception, allowing him to make his own decisions free from these autonomy-compromising influences. Given this, it was held that a negligent healthcare provider could respect her patient's autonomy provided that she refrained from subjecting him to these influences. This claim, however, can be challenged. While it is plausible to hold that a person, A, with no particular duties towards another person, B, could respect her autonomy simply by refraining from interfering in her decisions and actions it is not clear that the same could be said of A if he had certain duties incumbent upon him to treat B in particular ways. Thus, if by virtue of his particular relationship with B, A was duty-bound to help B enhance the instrumental value of his autonomy, if A negligently failed to do this he would be culpable for this failure—and culpable on the basis that he failed to respond appropriately to B's autonomy.[28] It is clear that healthcare professionals have duties towards their patients that arise from their professional association. Moreover, it is plausible to believe that one of these duties is for healthcare professionals to ensure that they aid their patients to enhance the instrumental value of their autonomy by working to aid them to secure or improve their health. (As was noted in Chapter 6 in the context of discussing kidney sales from live vendors, for many persons' ill health will reduce the instrumental value of their autonomy to them.) As such, then, even though it is plausible to believe that *typically* one person would respect the autonomy of another simply by failing to interfere with her, it is also plausible to believe that the professional duties of healthcare providers require that they respect their patients' autonomy not merely by failing to interfere with them in autonomy-compromising ways but by actively working to enhance the instrumental value of their autonomy to them in ways that are morally required by their professional standing.[29] Given this, then, it is possible to hold that a healthcare provider who negligently failed to secure the informed consent of her patients to their treatment *is* morally culpable for this, on the grounds that she failed appropriately to respect their autonomy. The above argument against the conventional understanding of the relationship between autonomy and informed consent thus fails. In focusing solely on the fact that a negligent healthcare provider would not act to compromise the autonomy of her patients' simpliciter (i.e., her negligence did not render them less autonomous with respect to their consequent decisions and actions), it fails to recognize that healthcare professionals have duties concerning the instrumental value of their patients' autonomy that extend beyond those that are incumbent upon persons who lack this relationship to others. As such, then, the conventional understanding of the relationship between autonomy and informed consent is defensible. Given that healthcare providers owe their patients a duty to secure or enhance the instrumental value of their autonomy to them through securing or enhancing their health, then, the ethical foundation of the doctrine of informed consent can be seen to be concern for the instrumental value of personal autonomy.[30]

## CONCLUSION

The received opinion among both medical ethicists and the legal profession is that the ethical foundation of the doctrine of informed consent is concern for autonomy. As with the received wisdom concerning the relationship between patient autonomy and patient confidentiality, there is, however, a paucity of arguments offered to establish autonomy as the ethical foundation of informed consent. And, as the arguments in this chapter showed, this omission is troublesome, for if one focuses on negligent failures to secure patients' informed consent it appears that concern for autonomy cannot play this foundational role. Despite this, however, once the argumentative emphasis is shifted from focusing on the protection of persons' autonomy itself to the duties that healthcare providers have to secure or enhance the *instrumental* value of their patients' autonomy for them it becomes clear how concern for autonomy can justify a concern with securing patients' informed consent. As with the conclusion of the last chapter, however, this defense of the conventional view of the relationship between autonomy and informed consent shows that this relationship is not as direct as it is usually believed. Indeed, as will be argued in the next chapter, the arguments in both this chapter and Chapter 8 support the view that autonomy is of primarily instrumental, rather than intrinsic, value—a conclusion that might come as a surprise to many who draw on this concept in bioethics.

# 10  The Value of Autonomy in Bioethics

## INTRODUCTION

It is clear from the previous discussions in this volume that autonomy has instrumental value; it is this that justified the claim that a valuer of autonomy should prefer that persons have more choices rather than fewer, as well as justifying concern for both the maintenance of patient confidentiality and securing patients' informed consent to their treatments.[1] But noting that autonomy is of instrumental value leads immediately to the question of what further value it is instrumental in securing. From the discussions in Chapters 6, 8, and 9, it seems clear that the best candidate for the value that autonomy is instrumental in securing is that of enabling persons to act to attempt to satisfy their own desires and secure their own goals. It was argued in Chapter 6 that a valuer of autonomy should prefer that persons have more choices rather than fewer because in such a situation persons would be more likely to be able to exercise their autonomy to satisfy their own desires or achieve their own goals. Similarly, in Chapter 8 it was argued that patient confidentiality should be respected because doing so would be more likely than the alternative to create a situation in which persons could exercise their autonomy effectively to achieve these ends, while in Chapter 9 it was argued that healthcare professionals should secure their patients' informed consent to their treatment on the grounds that this would be most likely to facilitate their using their autonomy in this way. This is, of course, a fairly loose account of what the value that autonomy is instrumental in securing is. However, without further analysis of the value of enabling such act-attempts it would be unwise to speculate further as to how this should be more precisely characterized. It might, for example, be that it transpires that the value that the exercise of autonomy is instrumental in securing is that of human well-being.[2] Alternatively, it might be that autonomy is instrumentally valuable in securing such act-attempts as part of a eudaimonistic human life (where the understanding of this concept is not reducible to an analysis of well-being), or that these act-attempts are simply valuable in their own right.

Autonomy, then, is clearly of instrumental value in contemporary medical settings. But is it also of *intrinsic* value?[3] It will be argued in this chapter that it is not. However, before moving to consider the arguments for the view that it is, and then on to the arguments against holding autonomy to be of intrinsic value, it should be noted that holding that autonomy is not of intrinsic value does not preclude a person from valuing autonomy for its own sake. A person might, for example, rationally prefer to make her own decisions and direct her own actions even though she recognizes that in doing so less of her desires would be satisfied and less of her goals achieved than would be were she to abdicate her self-direction to another. This preference would be rational for this person insofar as she also had a preference to exercise her autonomy for its own sake, and not merely for the sake of satisfying her other preferences. She would thus be willing to trade off the satisfaction of some of her preferences to satisfy her preference that her preferences be satisfied (if at all) though her own autonomous efforts.[4] Yet since such a person would prefer to exercise her autonomy rather than have other of her preferences satisfied through abdicating her effective decision-making over how she should act to another, in so doing she would indeed be satisfying (at least one of) her preferences and achieving (at least one of) her goals. As such, then, the value of such a person's autonomy to her would still be derivative from the value to her of fulfilling her preferences and achieving her goals.

## HURKA'S ARGUMENT FOR THE INTRINSIC VALUE OF AUTONOMY

It is often claimed that personal autonomy is of intrinsic value. Marilyn Friedman, for example, simply (and boldly) asserts that "Personal autonomy has intrinsic value," and this mantra is repeated frequently throughout both the literature on autonomy and the literature on bioethics.[5] Unfortunately, not only are few arguments presented in favor of this view but those that are presented fail. And this should not be surprising, for there is good reason to believe that it is false.

One prominent argument for the view that autonomy is intrinsically valuable has been developed by Thomas Hurka. Hurka argues that autonomy is intrinsically valuable insofar as autonomous agents more fully realize the ideal of causally efficacious agency, "of making a causal impact on the world and determining facts about it".[6] This is because, argues Hurka, when a person chooses among a set of options and chooses option *a*, she not only makes *a* the case, she also makes it the case that the other options are not chosen: that is, she makes it the case that not-*b*, not-*c*, not-*d*, and so on.[7] If, however, a person only had choice *a* available to her she would determine fewer facts about the world, and so be less "expansively an agent."[8]

There is, however, a fundamental objection to Hurka's argument: that even if it is correct it does not show that *autonomy* is of intrinsic value but only that *an agent's having choices* is. To be sure, for Hurka, all that is required for an agent to be autonomous is that she choose among options, where such choice might simply consist of an agent picking blindly from among those that are available to her.[9] (Hurka accepts that even though it would be better were an agent to deliberate about her options for this "gives her more intentions in and around her options than if she had picked blindly among them . . . ," and this would enhance "even further her agency," such deliberation is not necessary for an agent to be autonomous on his conception of autonomy.)[10] But, as was argued in Chapter 7, this conception of autonomy on which an agent is autonomous if it picks without interference from a range of options presented to it is too minimal to warrant the name, for such picking need not involve the self-direction that is the hallmark of autonomy. (Indeed, Hurka implicitly concedes this when he accepts that he is reducing autonomy to agency.)[11] As such, then, Hurka is not concerned with arguing directly for the intrinsic value of autonomy but for the intrinsic value of agency. To note this is not, however, also to note that Hurka's argument is not an argument for the view that autonomy is intrinsically valuable. This is because since autonomous agents are agents, then, if the exercise of agency is intrinsically valuable, the exercise of autonomy would also be intrinsically valuable insofar as it would be an instantiation of this. Hurka's argument, then, should be understood as an *indirect* argument for the intrinsic value of autonomy.

Yet even when Hurka's argument is understood in this way it is unconvincing.

Claudia Mills has noted that "surely it cannot be a particularly valuable exercise of agency simply to bring about all the ways in which the world is not, to be responsible for determining a myriad of things that are not the case," for "not all the not-doings we effect are morally substantive."[12] Mills acknowledges that Hurka attempts to meet this objection by distinguishing between the not-doings that persons effect that are important, and which enhance their agency, and the not-doings that are of minimal value, by distinguishing between deliberate choices whose choosers "choose goals which organize and encompass many others subordinate to them in a means-end hierarchy" and those that do not.[13] Hurka's example of the former type of choice is of choosing "to complete a year-long programme of self-improvement," while his example of the latter type of choice is of lifting a fork.[14] Against this attempted distinction Mills holds that "there are simply too many ways that the world is not for us to be able even to differentiate them, let alone to see them as flowing from our own casual powers . . . ," and, as such, "Claims about the significance of our choosing not to do things cannot bear the weight Hurka seeks to place on them."[15]

It is not clear, however, how Mills's objection to Hurka's argument is supposed to work. It could be understood as an epistemological objection, charging that we cannot determine in which respects the world is *not* a certain way flow from our choices. But if this is the case then Hurka seems to have a ready response: that whether or not we can tell how effective our causal powers are in making the world a certain way the fact remains that some of our choices will bring it about that the world is not a certain way to a greater extent than others, and since this is so our being able to have this negative effect on the world is intrinsically important. Drawing from this possible response that Hurka could offer, however, shows that Mills's objection to his argument for the intrinsic value of autonomy should be understood as an ontological one: that, contra Hurka, it is not clear that it is possible to differentiate the negative effects of our choices in the way that he believes. To develop Mills's objection, this is because the negative ramifications of all our actions will stretch far into the future, and, as such, it is not clear that those choices that Hurka believes to be significant would have any greater negative effects (i.e., not-doings) in the long run than those that he considers to be insignificant.

Hurka's argument for the view that autonomy is intrinsically valuable is also subject to a further objection: that it is not clear why an agent's having a causal effect on the world is itself intrinsically valuable. It is not clear, for example, why it is *intrinsically* valuable that a person who chooses a career as a teacher does so from a range of options, and, in doing so, makes it the case that she does not become, for example, a lawyer, a politician, or an accountant.[16] To be sure, such a person would be responsible for a greater number of negative facts about her life than someone who only had the option of becoming a teacher available to her. Yet it is not clear why *this* is intrinsically valuable—and, given that Hurka's argument is aimed primarily at showing that the exercise of such agency is intrinsically valuable this question needs to be addressed directly. Indeed, it would seem that a better explanation as to why being able to choose from a range of possible careers rather than just one is that in doing so a person is more likely to have a career that she is suited to. But this shows that a person's exercise of autonomy is not of intrinsic value, as Hurka claims, but of *instrumental* value, in that (as outlined previously), its exercise will be likely to enable her to satisfy her preferences or achieve her goals.

## AGAINST THE VIEW THAT AUTONOMY HAS INTRINSIC VALUE

### Arguments From Covert Manipulation and Covert Surveillance

Hurka, then, has failed to show that autonomy has intrinsic value. And, moreover, there seems to be a good reason to believe that it does not. It is clear from the discussion of Iago's manipulation of Othello in Chapter 1, and the subsequent and related discussions in Chapters 3, 8, and 9, that for one person to exert control over another she must intend to do so. With this point in hand, consider a third version of *Othello*. In this version of the play Iago, while just as cunning and manipulative as he was in the original version, is absentminded, and sometimes forgets that he is trying to manipulate Othello to do as he wishes. Absentminded Iago thus vacillates between the situation of Iago in the original play and the unmanipulative McIago of *McOthello*. When he is in the same situation as the original Iago (i.e., he is intending to manipulate Othello and is successful in doing so), Othello will suffer from a diminution in his autonomy with respect to his decisions and his actions. When he is in the same situation as McIago, however (i.e., he is not intending to manipulate Othello but provides him with the same information as the original Iago did, with the same results), Othello will not suffer from any diminution in his autonomy at all.[17] As such, then, Othello will vacillate between being fully autonomous with respect to his decisions and actions and suffering from compromised autonomy with respect to them, depending upon the mental states of Absentminded Iago. But, since Othello's decisions and actions will be the same whether he is autonomous with respect to them or not, and since they will have precisely the same effects, it seems that it should not matter to Othello whether or not he enjoys autonomy with respect to them. As such, then, it seems that in this situation Othello should be indifferent as to whether or not he was autonomous with respect to his decisions and actions—and this would not be the case were his autonomy to be of intrinsic value. A similar example with the same conclusion can be drawn from the conclusions of Chapter 8. The arguments presented there showed that a person will suffer from a diminution in his autonomy with respect to his decisions and actions if (provided the four conditions outlined in that chapter were met) he is placed under covert surveillance. With this point in hand, consider two worlds. In World One P is placed under covert surveillance in a situation in which the four additional conditions outlined in Chapter 8 are met; in World Two he is not. Other than this, however, P's life in World One is identical to his life in World Two; he makes the same decisions, has and satisfies the same desires, performs the same actions, and experiences precisely the same amount of pleasures and pains in both Worlds. Since this is so, it seems plausible to claim that since the diminution of P's autonomy in World One had no effect on his life, it does not matter that P has suffered this loss. Hence, then, like that of Othello, P's autonomy is not valuable for its own sake. Thus, if it does not matter that either Othello or P suffer from diminutions in their autonomy, then even though autonomy might be of instrumental value to the persons who possess it, it is not valuable for its own sake.

## Nozick's Experience Machine and Feinberg's Case A

However, this argument against the view that autonomy has intrinsic value might move too quickly. This is because it relies upon the hedonistic assumption that only events that persons experience can affect their lives, and so if an event does not affect a person's experiences then it cannot affect her life in any way. But this assumption can be challenged. If it were true that only events that persons experience can affect their lives, then there would be nothing to choose between living a real life and living a life plugged into a machine that would simulate exactly the same experiences as would be had by the person living the real life. Moreover, if the experiences in the life lived in the machine to be more pleasurable than those that would be had by living the real life, then, were this hedonistic assumption to be true, one should prefer to live the simulated life rather than the real life.[18] Thus, if even when the experiences in the simulated life are more pleasurable than those in the real life, the real life transpires to be preferable to its simulated counterpart, it is clear that something other than a person's experiences can affect her life. Turning back to the examples of Othello and P, then, if Nozick's conclusions concerning such an experience machine are correct we could judge that the play in which Othello was most autonomous is preferable to the others, and that World One could be preferable to World Two for P. And since this is so, we could judge that autonomy is valuable for its own sake, even if its possession otherwise makes no difference to the life of its possessor.

In a similar vein Joel Feinberg argues against the hedonistic assumption that underlies the previous argument against the view that autonomy is intrinsically valuable, holding that "the area of a person's good or harm is necessarily wider than his subjective interest. . ."[19] In support of this Feinberg, following W. D. Ross, distinguishes between want-fulfillment and want-satisfaction.[20] When a want is *fulfilled* that which was wanted comes into existence; when a want is *satisfied* the person who had the want experiences gratification or contentment as a result of this. With this distinction in place, Feinberg holds that "Most persons will agree. . .that the important thing is to get what they want, even if that causes no joy," for "the object of our efforts is to fulfill our wants in the external world, not to bring about states of our own minds."[21] Thus, concludes Feinberg, the thwarting of a person's interests will harm him even if he never learns that this has occurred—just as their fulfillment will benefit him even if he never learns of this. To support this, Feinberg has developed the following example:

> Case A: A woman devotes thirty years of her life to the furtherance of certain ideals and ambitions in the form of one vast undertaking. She founds an institution dedicated to these ends and works single-mindedly for its advancement, both for the sake of the social good she believes it to promote, and for the sake of her own glory. One month before she dies, the "empire of her hopes" collapses utterly as the establishment into which she has poured her life's energies crumbles into ruin, and she is personally disgraced. She never learns the unhappy truth, however, as her friends, eager to save her from disappointment, conceal or misrepresent the facts. She dies contented.[22]

Feinberg notes that, "It would not be very controversial to say that the woman in Case A had suffered grievous harm to her interests although she never learned the bad news."[23] Since this is so, the hedonistic assumption that underlay the argument, given previously, against the view that autonomy was intrinsically valuable (that only events that a person experiences can affect her life), seems to be mistaken, for even though the collapse of this woman's "empire of her hopes" never affects her experiences it does harm her. Thus, if Othello had an interest in being maximally autonomous with respect to his desires and his actions, then the mental states that Absentminded Iago had *would* make a difference to him even if they would make no difference either to the actions that he performed or to his experiences. This is because Absentminded Iago's possession of certain mental states (i.e., those aimed at manipulating Othello) would (when combined with the appropriate and successful manipulative actions) lead to the thwarting of this interest of Othello's. Similarly, given P's interests, it would make a difference to him as to whether he was in World One or World Two, for he would be harmed in World One in a way that he would not be in World Two. However, since both Othello and P would perform the same actions and have the same experiences irrespective of whether they are manipulated or placed under covert surveillance, it does not matter with respect to the instrumental value of their autonomy whether they were manipulated or placed under surveillance. As such, then, since, given their interests it *would* matter to them whether they were manipulated or placed under surveillance or not, their autonomy must be valuable to them for its own sake. Thus, not only does the previous argument against the view that autonomy is of intrinsic value seem to fail, but the objections to it seem to show that autonomy is of intrinsic value after all.

## Responding to the Nozickian Argument

The Nozickian response to the prior argument against the view that autonomy has intrinsic value is certainly persuasive. However, it can be undermined by considering it in connection with Berkeley's view that the universe consists solely of ideas.[24] Like persons in the experience machine, persons in a Berkeleyian universe will have contact only with ideas. They will, essentially, live within an experience machine of God's making. Moreover, the Berkeleyian universe will be no different experientially from the universe that we inhabit now. (Indeed, this universe might well *be* a Berkeleyian universe!) Since this is so, there seems to be no reason to object to entering into an experience machine, especially if the experiences that one would have within it would be more pleasurable than those that would be had without it. After all, if the actual universe could be (effectively) an experience machine, and yet the lives lived within it do not, contra the implication of Nozick's experience machine argument, lack anything, then the mere fact that the experience machine *is* an experience machine should make no difference to one. Since there is thus nothing to choose between the "real" world and the experience machine, Nozick's claim that intuitively there is something to choose between the "real" world and the experience machine turns out to be mistaken. And since it is this claim that supports the view that something besides a person's experiences (such as, for example, whether her interests were fulfilled) will play a role in determining how well her life goes, Nozick has given us no reason to reject the hedonistic intuition that underlay the previous argument against the view that personal autonomy is intrinsically valuable.

One might, however, attempt to respond to this Berkeleyian argument by claiming that there is an important difference between the experience machine and a Berkeleyian universe: that the persons within the experience machine are deceived about how well their lives are going, since their experiences do not reflect how the world really is, whereas the inhabitants of a Berkeleyian world are not so deceived, for they have access to the only reality possible. But this response would be unsatisfactory. First, in assuming that being subject to deception is bad for the persons within the experience machine, that is, that their being deceived makes their lives worse than those of the persons outside the machine, this objection begs the question against the hedonist assumption.[25] To argue against this assumption it cannot simply be assumed that the life of a person whose experiences are the product of deception is thereby worse than that of a person whose identical experiences are not the product of deception; this must be shown. Second, to place persons into the experience machine is not obviously to subject them to deception at all; it simply is to create a new world for them.[26] To see this, consider a universe in which there is not merely one God, but many demi-gods, each of was created by God, and each of which creates and sustains neo-Berkeleyian universes for their creatures. Such demi-gods would not be deceiving their creatures in so doing; they would simply be providing them with their existences and worlds in which to live them out. Now consider a slightly different situation; God is the sole creature creator, and yet it is open to the demi-gods to secure His other creatures and to place them in worlds of their creation. Again, it seems that to do so would not be to subject such creatures to deception; it would merely be to have them live their lives in a world created and sustained by one supernatural being rather than another. As such, then, were the "superduper neurosurgeons" of Nozick's example to be considered to be such demi-gods, they would not be deceiving their subjects, but, instead, would simply be creating new worlds for them to live in.

## Responding to Feinberg's Argument

Nozick's example of the experience machine, then, gives us no reason to believe that how well a person's life goes is determined by anything other than her experiences. It thus gives us no reason to believe that Othello would have any reason to prefer being in *McOthello* rather than the original *Othello* or the *Othello* with Absentminded Iago, or that World One is preferable to P than World Two. What, then, of Feinberg's Case A? Like Nozick's example of the experience machine Case A is supposed to show that even if an event has no effect on a person's experiences it can still affect how well her life goes by thwarting her interests. If this is so, then there could be reason for Othello to choose *McOthello* over the other variants of *Othello*, or for P to prefer World One to World Two—and so the previous argument against the view that autonomy is of intrinsic value would fail.

The force of Feinberg's Case A rests on his claim that it is not "very controversial" to hold that the woman whose empire of hopes collapsed was harmed by this. But closer examination of this example should undermine Feinberg's confidence here. Three views are generated by this example: (i) that if the woman's project is of social worth, it is bad that it collapsed; (ii) that the woman was harmed by the deception of her friends simply in virtue of being deceived; and (iii) that the woman was harmed by the collapse of her project even though this never affected her experiences.[27] The first of these views is irrelevant to the question of whether the woman herself was harmed, for the failure of her project might be bad for others (e.g., its intended beneficiaries) while not being bad for her. Views (ii) and (iii) are distinct, but both support Feinberg's view that a person can be harmed by an event even if it does not affect her life. It is clear that view (ii) on its own cannot be used to support the anti-hedonistic argument against the view that autonomy is not intrinsically valuable, for unless it receives argumentative support to use it for this purpose would be to beg the question. As such, then, the focus must be on view (iii) to show that Case A does not support the anti-hedonistic intuition.

The simplest way to undermine Feinberg's view that the conclusions that he wishes to draw from Case A are not "very controversial" is to construct an example that is directly analogous to this Case, but which clearly does not support view (iii). In this regard consider a woman who in her youth planted some cypress trees and who wishes that they live to a great age. She has retained this interest throughout her life and is now in a nursing home, unable to visit her trees but confident that they are flourishing. Unfortunately, they have sickened and died. The woman has no one to tell her of the fate of her trees, and she dies content, believing them to be doing well. Does the death of these trees harm this woman? Intuitively, it seems that it does not, even though her interest in their well-being has been thwarted. On its own, however, this revised version of Case A—the "Cypress Case"—is unpersuasive, for it begs the question against Feinberg, who could simply respond by insisting that insofar as this woman's interests in her trees were thwarted then she was harmed by their sickening and dying. Of course, one might try to bolster the intuitive force of the Cypress Case by stipulating that the trees die centuries after the woman's death, and that her interest was that they lived on in perpetuity. Yet while this revised version of the Cypress Case might be more intuitively persuasive (are, for example, long-dead Egyptian pharaohs really harmed by the excavation of their tombs, even though they made it clear that they had an interest in remaining undisturbed?),[28] Feinberg could still respond by claiming that the woman (and the pharaohs) are harmed by the thwarting of their interests, even though such thwarting will occur long after she (and they) is (and are) dead.[29] Moreover, there seems to be a second problem with the Cypress Case: that it is disanalogous to Case A insofar as in the latter case, but not the former, the woman in question could be said to be harmed as a result of the damage done to her reputation (i.e., as a successful philanthropist) through the collapse of her undertaking.

To undermine Feinberg's view that the conclusions that he wishes to draw from Case A are not "very controversial," then, it needs to be argued that there are good theoretical reasons for rejecting his claim that the woman in Case A was harmed by the collapse of her enterprises. To begin to argue against Feinberg in this way it should be noted that Feinberg develops Case A in the context of arguing that posthumous harm is possible—that is, that persons can be harmed while they are alive by events that occur after their deaths that thwart their interests. Feinberg uses Case A in the context of this discussion to support the view (that is the target of criticism here) that persons can be harmed by events even if their experiences are not affected by them. With this Case in hand Feinberg develops Case B, in which the woman's undertaking collapses a year after her death.[30] Feinberg claims that since the woman's interests in Case B were thwarted to the same extent as they were in Case A, and since (he believes) it was correct to hold that the woman in Case A was harmed by this thwarting even though it did not affect her experiences, then the woman in Case B was harmed by the similar thwarting of her interests. Feinberg recognizes that there might be a problem with attributing harm to the woman in Case B insofar as it seems to require backwards causation, with the cause of her harm occurring later than its occurrence. To address this concern Feinberg draws on the work of George Pitcher, who argues that ascribing posthumous harms to persons need not commit one to endorsing the possibility of backwards causation.[31] This is because, argues Pitcher, ascriptions of posthumous harms to persons should be understood in the same way as ascribing such properties as penultimacy should be understood. If an event destroyed the world in the presidency of the president of the United States who served after Ronald Reagan, this would make it true that Reagan was the penultimate president of the United States, but such an ascription of this property to him would not commit one to endorsing backwards causation.[32]

Feinberg, then, is willing to accept that his anti-hedonistic view that a person is harmed when her interests are thwarted commits him to holding that posthumous harm is possible—and he is willing to defend this latter claim. Given this, if it can be shown that there is reason to reject the Feinberg–Pitcher view that posthumous harm is possible, and since this view is one that Feinberg is committed to given his claims in Case A, then the rejection of the possibility of posthumous harm will show that Feinberg's anti-hedonistic Case A should be rejected also. And if this is so then we will have no reason to believe that Othello would have any reason to prefer being in *McOthello* rather than the original *Othello* or the *Othello* with Absentminded Iago, or that World One is preferable to P than World Two. And if *this* is so then the hedonistic assumption that only events that persons experience can affect their lives that undergirds the previous argument against the view that autonomy has intrinsic value will be defensible against the prior objections to it. And there *is* reason to reject the Feinberg–Pitcher view that posthumous harm is possible, for Pitcher's defense of the claim that endorsing posthumous harm need not commit one to endorsing backwards causation is flawed. "Penultimacy" is a sequential property; it is a property that something will possess in virtue of being located at a particular point in a sequence. "Harm," however, is not a sequential property but one that is ascribed to a person (roughly) if an event results in his well being being lower than it was (or would have been) prior to the event (or than it would have been had the event not occurred).[33]

Thus, while Pitcher is correct to note that facts after a person's death could result in sequential properties being ascribed to her, this does not support his claim that *harms* could similarly be ascribed to persons on the basis of events that occur after their deaths. Since Pitcher has failed to make his case for the view that endorsing posthumous harm need not commit one to endorsing backwards causation it seems that the Feinberg–Pitcher account of posthumous harm is wedded to this metaphysically dubious notion—and so is itself metaphysically dubious.[34] As such, then, since Feinberg's anti-hedonistic account of harm (supported by Cases A and B) commits him to holding that posthumous harm is possible, there is reason to reject it. There is thus reason also to reject the previous objections to the hedonistic assumption that only events that persons experience can affect their lives that undergirds the previous argument against the view that autonomy has intrinsic value.

What, then, of the second problem with the Cypress Case outlined previously: that it is disanalogous to Feinberg's Case A insofar as it writes out the possibility that the woman in question is the victim of reputational harm? The immediate response to this second objection might be that it is now moot. This is because the previous response to the Feinberg–Pitcher defense of the possibility of posthumous harm shows that Feinberg's anti-hedonistic, interest-based, account of well-being that is supported by Case A should not be accepted—and so there is no reason to believe that the thwarting of a woman's interests in her reputation will in itself be a harm to her. But this immediate response to the previous concern about reputational harm is too quick, for the possibility of reputational harm could be used to defend the Feinberg–Pitcher view that posthumous harm is possible. And if this defense is successful, then there would be, once again, reason to reject the hedonistic assumption that undergirds the previous argument against the view that autonomy has intrinsic value.

It was argued previously that the Feinberg–Pitcher account of how posthumous harm is possible should be rejected for, despite Pitcher's arguments to the contrary, it still seems to be committed to the possibility of backwards causation. The notion of reputational harm might, however, provide a way to show how harms—and not just sequential properties— could be ascribed to persons after their deaths. On the counterfactual account of harm that was developed previously a person is harmed by an event E if it results in his well-being being lower than it was (or would have been) prior to E (or than it would have been had the E not occurred). The proponents of this counterfactual account of harm will accept that a person could be harmed by a loss provided that it would leave him worse off than he would have been had it not occurred. And persons can, it seems at first sight, lose things after their deaths. As Barbara Baum Levenbook argues, the assumption that such losses are possible "cannot be rejected on the grounds that there is no loser to do the losing . . . . Einstein has not lost his reputation as a scientific genius, even though he had that reputation until his death. One must claim either that he cannot lose it now, having retained the reputation until his death and now being incapable of losing anything, or that he still has the reputation and can lose it now."[35] Thus, if Einstein could lose his reputation now, and this loss would adversely affect his well-being, then it seems that posthumous harm is possible. And, if this is so, then the anti-hedonistic conclusion of Feinberg's Case A could be resurrected and used to undermine the previous argument against the view that autonomy has intrinsic value.

But there are two serious difficulties with using the notion of reputational harm to resurrect the Feinberg–Pitcher account of posthumous harm in this way. First, this argument illegitimately presupposes that were Einstein to lose his reputation postmortem this would adversely affect his well-being while he was alive. But, since the whole point of this use of the possibility of reputational harm is to show that a person could be harmed (i.e., that his well-being would be adversely affected) by the postmortem loss of his reputation this presupposition simply begs the question. Second, as Joan Callahan notes, it is simply not true to say that Einstein could lose his reputation after his death, except in a purely figurative sense. This is because, she argues, claims about Einstein's reputation are not claims about something that *Einstein* has but claims about the mental states of persons who have beliefs about Einstein.[36] Thus, claims about reputational harms, benefits, or losses are simply claims about the mental states of persons who have beliefs about the subjects of these reputations and so such claims about reputations cannot be sued to support claims about posthumous harms, benefits, or losses. Moreover, Callahan notes, since Einstein does not exist there really is no subject to bear the loss that Levenbook ascribes to him.[37]

Once the strands of intuition that surround Case A have been teased apart, then, and it has been reformed so that it will directly support (iii) only, it fails to do so. Like Nozick's example of the experience machine, then, Feinberg's Case A fails to show that something other than a person's experiences can affect how well her life goes. It thus cannot be used to undermine the previous argument for the view that autonomy is not of intrinsic value, for if it does not show that something other than a person's experiences determine how well her life goes it cannot be used to show that Othello should prefer to be in the play in which he enjoyed the greatest degree of autonomy, or that P should prefer to be in World One rather than World Two.

## A Third Response

With this discussion of Nozick's example of the experience machine and Feinberg's Case A in hand in the context of a discussion of the issue of whether or not there is a reason to believe that autonomy is of intrinsic value a simpler argument for the view that it is not should not be overlooked. Recall here Dworkin's argument, discussed in Chapter 6, that a person's having fewer choices is not necessarily worse for her than her having more.[38] Dworkin's argument for this conclusion was based on the claim that it would be irrational for a person to choose to have two of his lesser-ranked options in preference to having only his highest rank option to choose from. While Dworkin's claim here is subject to criticism, the general form of his argument can be applied to the cases of Othello and P, given previously. Thus, in considering these cases one could simply ask whether it is plausible to hold that Othello would prefer to be in the play with McIago rather than with Iago or Absentminded Iago, given that it would make no difference to how he lived his life? Similarly, one could ask whether it is plausible to hold that P would have any preferences between World One and World Two, given that he, too, would be unable to detect any difference between them? It seems likely that it would not be plausible to hold that these people would have these preferences—and since the only reason that they would, would be if they held autonomy to have intrinsic value, it seems plausible to maintain that autonomy is not valuable in this way. Of course, it is open for a defender of the view that autonomy is intrinsically valuable to assert that were *she* to be in the position of Othello or P *she* would prefer to be in the play with McIago, and she would prefer to be World One. But to make sense of this apparently puzzling claim to others such a defender of the view that autonomy is intrinsically valuable would have to provide reasons for her choices. And, given that Hurka's argument for this position has already been undermined it is not obvious what form such reasons would take.

## AUTONOMY AND BIOETHICAL PUBLIC POLICY

If the value of personal autonomy is instrumental this will have important implications for discussions of political liberalism. The alleged intrinsic value of autonomy is often taken to ground various restrictions on what states should and should not do. It is, for example, taken to support proscriptions against paternalism,[39] to protect freedom of speech,[40] and to require state neutrality towards differing conceptions of the good.[41] All of these autonomy-based restrictions on state action have implications for public policy as this pertains to bioethical issues. They would, for example, militate against the paternalistic recommendations outlined in the United Kingdom Government's white paper on public health, *Choosing Health*,[42] justify protecting speech advertising the availability of abortions in states where they are legal,[43] or pharmacists advertising the prices of prescription drugs,[44] and require that states not privilege one approach to the patient–physician relationship over another where the differing approaches in question are the result of different cultural expectations.[45] Given this, it might appear at first sight that if the value of autonomy is instrumental these bulwarks against state interference in persons' medical decisions would vanish, or, at the very least, be weakened. But this is not so. As was noted by Smith, given the fact of value pluralism respecting the *instrumental* value of autonomy in framing public policy is important precisely because this is a way to ensure that the ability of individual citizens to pursue their own interests within a pluralistic polity is protected.[46] Moreover, focusing on the protection of individual's abilities to act as they wish within a pluralistic society through focusing on respecting the instrumental value of their autonomy to them is likely to provide a *stronger* bulwark against a state's interference in medical choices of its citizens (and, indeed, in their lives in general) than would a focus on the (alleged) *intrinsic* value of autonomy. To see this, consider Hurka's claim that "To violate a citizen's autonomy the state need not try forcing her into one best activity. Instead of removing all but one of ten options it may remove just the bottom two, on the ground that they are intrinsically bad. This more limited coercion—forbidding the worst rather than requiring the best . . . still (somewhat) reduces autonomy."[47] However, as was argued in Chapter 6, to remove two options from a person's choice-set does *not*, contra Hurka, "violate" a person's autonomy at all.[48] At most, it will make its exercise *less instrumentally valuable* for her. If one is concerned with autonomy simpliciter, then, one should have no objection to states removing options from persons' choice-sets in this way, by, for example, prohibiting the sale of certain pharmaceuticals. If, however, one is concerned with the instrumental value of personal autonomy then one should *prima facie* object to the state's removal of such options on the grounds that to do so is illegitimately to prejudge which options would create value for persons if they chose them. A concern for the instrumental value of personal autonomy could thus justify greater restrictions upon state activity than could a concern with the intrinsic value of autonomy.

To focus on the value to persons of the exercise of their autonomy is, however, a double-edged sword for persons concerned with justifying restricting states' interferences in the medical choices (and lives in general) of their citizens. Just as a focus on the instrumental value of the exercise of personal autonomy to the persons exercising it could, as outlined previously, provide the basis for arguments that seek to restrict state actions (e.g., the state's removal of what it considers to be unpalatable options from persons' choice-sets, such as those afforded by current markets in human transplant kidneys), so too could it provide the basis for arguments that seek to *increase* the role of the state in the lives of its citizens. Noting that being in mired in poverty is likely to decrease the instrumental value of a person's exercise of autonomy to her (although being impoverished would not compromise her autonomy simpliciter), one could argue in favor of wealth redistribution. Here, one could argue that since the redistribution of resources away from the comparatively wealthy towards the impoverished would not significantly reduce their ability to exercise their autonomy, but it *is* likely greatly to enhance the ability of the impoverished to exercise theirs, concern for the instrumental value of the exercise of autonomy justifies such redistribution.[49] Yet despite the initial plausibility of such an argument it might be too glib. To compare in this way the ability of different persons to exercise their autonomy obscures the fact that the value of such exercise is (at least with respect to the obvious instrumental value that autonomy possesses) derivative from the value to persons of their being enabled to satisfy their preferences or achieve their goals. As such, while focusing on interpersonal comparisons of exercises of autonomy might appear to be straightforward in that instances of the exercise of the same capacity are being compared, it is not, for the instrumental value of a person's exercise of her autonomy is derivative from the degree of preference satisfaction or goal achievement that such exercise enables her to accomplish. As such, then, interpersonal comparisons of the value of differing exercises of autonomy are subject to the same difficulties that interpersonal comparisons of preference satisfaction and goal achievements are subject to.[50] And recognizing this should lead to greater, rather than fewer, restrictions being placed upon states' interferences in the medical choices of their citizens.


## CONCLUSION

The arguments in this chapter are the natural culmination of the earlier discussions in this volume of the relationships that hold between the value of autonomy and the availability of choice, the value of autonomy and the concern for patient confidentiality, and the value of autonomy and the concern with securing patients' informed consent to their treatments. As was intimated in those discussions the value of autonomy within contemporary discussions of bioethical issues is instrumental, rather than intrinsic, such that it is valued for the advantages that its exercise can bring to those who possess it. The view that autonomy is implicitly accorded only instrumental value within bioethical discussions was supported in this chapter both by making more explicit the concerns that underlay the previous discussions and also by arguing that there is good reason to believe that the value of autonomy is not intrinsic. Recognizing this is helpful, not only because of the conceptual clarity that it could bring to discussions of contemporary bioethical issues in which the concept of autonomy plays a central role, but also because this recognition can be used to justify greater limitations on third-party interference in persons' medical choices. And this increased focus on the individual patient is a consummation devoutly to be wished.

# Conclusion

It is now time to take stock. It was noted in the Introduction to this volume
that autonomy is widely held to be the preeminent value in contemporary
bioethics. With this point in hand an account of practical autonomy was
developed with the explicit aim of capturing the contours of this concept
as it is used throughout the philosophical literature, from the foundational
theoretical discussions of autonomy theorists to the use of this concept
within moral philosophy, in general, and bioethics, in particular. Having developed this capturing account of practical autonomy it was argued
that, rather than its taking its place as merely one further conception of
autonomy among many, it should be recognized that there are not as many
extant accounts of autonomy proper as it might at first appear. As such,
then, it was argued, since it successfully captures the connotative contours
of this concept the account of practical autonomy developed in this volume
could legitimately lay claim to being one of the (if not *the*) core analyses of
autonomy that should be drawn on in discussions of this concept. Moreover, it was argued in this context that, despite their widespread conflation,
the concepts of autonomy and identification are distinct, with the former
being a *political* concept and the latter being a *metaphysical* one. Since
this is so, the defeating conditions for ascriptions of autonomy to persons
with respect to their decisions and consequent actions would be externally
orientated, focusing on the question of whether they, or someone else, were
in control of them. This account of practical autonomy is thus a radically
*externalist* account of autonomy, such that the question of whether a person is autonomous with respect to her decisions and actions will turn, in
part, on questions concerning the mental states of others. By contrast, the
defeating conditions for an account of identification would be internally
orientated, focusing on the relationships that held between the mental
states of the person whose identification with her desires is in question and
the genesis of her effective first-order desires.

Recognizing both that practical autonomy is a radically externalist concept
and that it is distinct from the concept of identification are, however, only the
first two striking claims that were argued for in this volume. It has also been
argued from this account of practical autonomy that a person who values

autonomy should, contra received philosophical wisdom, generally prefer that persons have more choices rather than fewer, and that, despite first appearances, this position is compatible with the view that a person's exercise of her autonomy is not only compatible with her being subject to constraints but actually *requires* this. And, as befits a discussion of *practical* autonomy, these two conclusions are not only of theoretical interest. That concern for the value of practical autonomy should lead one to prefer that persons have more choices rather than fewer should lead one to oppose public policies that are intended to restrict persons' choice-sets, such as laws prohibiting (or even highly regulating) current markets in human organs. Similarly, the recognition that a person's exercise of her practical autonomy need not be compromised by her being subject to constraint should lead one to recognize that persons who have been socialized into communitarian societies (such as the Amish), or women who have been socialized to accept norms that would be rejected by most feminists, or persons who have been socialized to accept metaphysical views that are not generally accepted (such as the Navajo's traditional view that speaking of possible misfortune will make it more likely to occur), do not thereby suffer from any diminutions in their autonomy, and so pose no special problem in this regard for bioethicists concerned with healthcare providers securing their patients' autonomous consent to their treatments.[1]

Just as it is clear that these theoretical conclusions concerning the relationships that hold among autonomy, choice, and constraint are striking in themselves and have interesting practical implications, so too is it clear that, as was argued in this volume, a correct understanding of practical autonomy (and hence a correct understanding of how it might be compromised) has striking implications for discussions of patient confidentiality and informed consent. But these implications are not, however, of only parochial interest to persons concerned with these particular issues. In showing *how* these concerns for patient confidentiality and securing patients' informed consent to their treatment are based on a concern for personal autonomy the discussion of these issues leads to a more general point: that implicit within many contemporary discussions of bioethical issues is the view that autonomy is of instrumental, rather than intrinsic, value. Recognizing this should also, like the two theoretical conclusions discussed previously, be of practical as well as theoretical interest, for (and unlike the view that autonomy is of *intrinsic* value) this view of the value of autonomy would support *prima facie* objections to the third-party removal of options from person's choice-sets—such as, for example, the option to sell a kidney. And this, of course, has immediate practical implications for many debates within both contemporary moral philosophy in general and bioethics in particular. At this point, then, it is clear that the promissory note that was issued in the Introduction to this volume—that a correct account of the concept of autonomy as this is understood within contemporary bioethics will serve to illuminate those discussions in which it plays a central role—has now been paid in full.

# Notes

## NOTES TO THE INTRODUCTION

1. It would take an entire volume to list all of the articles and books that recognize autonomy as being the preeminent value in contemporary Western bioethics. For representations of this view, however, see Janet Smith, "The Pre-eminence of Autonomy in Bioethics," in *Human Lives: Critical Essays on Consequentialist Bioethics,* eds. D. S. Oderberg and J. A. Laing, 182–195 (London/New York: Macmillan/St. Martin's Press, 1997); R. Gillon, "Ethics Needs Principles—Four Can Encompass the Rest—and Respect for Autonomy Should Be 'First Among Equals,'" *Journal of Medical Ethics* 29, no. 5 (2003): 307–312; and Henrik Levinsson, "Autonomy and Metacognition—A Healthcare Perspective" (PhD diss., Lund University, 2008), 3. It must be emphasized that persons who hold autonomy to be preeminent in bioethics do not thereby commit themselves to the view that its value is the only one pertinent to bioethical discussions; to do so would be, as James F. Childress has noted, to accept an "oversimplified, overextended, and overweighted" focus on the value of autonomy. See James F. Childress, "The Place of Autonomy in Bioethics," *Hastings Center Report* 20, no. 1 (1990): 12.
2. The distinction between Kantian autonomy and personal autonomy is outlined in James Stacey Taylor, "Introduction," in *Personal Autonomy: New Essays on Personal Autonomy and Its Role in Contemporary Moral Philosophy,* ed. James Stacey Taylor, 1 (Cambridge: Cambridge University Press, 2005).
3. Tom L. Beauchamp, "Who Deserves Autonomy, and Whose Autonomy Deserves Respect?" in *Personal Autonomy,* ed. Taylor, 327, n. 1.
4. John Christman, "Introduction," in *The Inner Citadel: Essays on Individual Autonomy,* ed. John Christman, 4 (New York: Oxford University Press, 1989).
5. H. Tristram Engelhardt Jr., *Foundations of Christian Bioethics* (Lisse, The Netherlands: Swets & Zeitlinger, 2000) 28. Engelhardt's views here are discussed in Jennifer Jackson, *Ethics in Medicine* (Cambridge: Polity Press, 2006), 64–67.
6. This approach is explicitly adopted in James Stacey Taylor, *Stakes and Kidneys,* in which it is noted that the arguments in that volume are conditional arguments only, directed only at persons who hold autonomy and well-being to be of moral importance. James Stacey Taylor, *Stakes and Kidneys: Why Markets in Human Body Parts are Morally Imperative* (Aldershot, England: Ashgate Publishing, 2005), 18.
7. Harry G. Frankfurt, "Freedom of the Will and the Concept of a Person," in *The Importance of What We Care About: Philosophical Essays,* ed. Harry

G. Frankfurt (Cambridge: Cambridge University Press, 1988), 11–25. Previously published in *The Journal of Philosophy* 68, no. 1 (1971): 5–20. (All further references to this essay will be to the reprinted version). In this essay Frankfurt was concerned with offering an account of what it is for a person to "identify" with her effective first-order desires, to act freely and of her own free will when she was moved by them. As will be argued in Chapter 3, the concept of identification is distinct from that of autonomy. Thus, even though it is true that Frankfurt's essay stimulated a great deal of philosophical interest in autonomy that it was taken to be an account of autonomy has also served to compromise the conceptual clarity of analyses of this concept. The burgeoning philosophical interest in autonomy is demonstrated by the publication of several important collections of papers and monographs that address it. See, for example, Robert Young, *Personal Autonomy: Beyond Negative and Positive Liberty* (London: Croom Helm Ltd, 1986); Christman, ed., *The Inner Citadel*; Frankfurt, ed., *The Importance of What We Care About* (Cambridge: Cambridge University Press, 1988); Gerald Dworkin, *The Theory and Practice of Autonomy* (Cambridge: Cambridge University Press, 1988); Keith Lehrer, *Metamind* (Oxford: Clarendon Press, 1990); Thomas Hill Jr., *Autonomy and Self-Respect* (Cambridge: Cambridge University Press, 1991); Diana Tietjens Meyers, *Self, Society, and Personal Choice* (New York: Columbia University Press, 1991); Alfred R. Mele, *Autonomous Agents: From Self-Control to Autonomy* (New York: Oxford University Press, 1995); Bernard Berofsky, *Liberation from Self: A Theory of Personal Autonomy* (Cambridge: Cambridge University Press, 1995); Carl E. Schneider, *The Practice of Autonomy: Patients, Doctors, and Medical Decisions* (New York: Oxford University Press, 1998); Harry G. Frankfurt, ed., *Necessity, Volition, and Love* (Cambridge: Cambridge University Press, 1999); Catriona Mackenzie and Natalie Stoljar, eds., *Relational Autonomy: Feminist Perspectives on Autonomy, Agency, and the Social Self* (Oxford: Oxford University Press, 2000); Stefaan E. Cuypers, *Self-Identity and Personal Autonomy* (Aldershot, England: Ashgate Publishing, 2002); Sarah Buss and Lee Overton, eds., *Contours of Agency: Essays on Themes from Harry Frankfurt* (Cambridge: MIT Press, 2003); Marilyn Friedman, *Autonomy, Gender, Politics* (New York: Oxford University Press, 2003); Ellen Frankel Paul, Fred D. Miller Jr., Jeffrey Paul, eds., *Autonomy* (Cambridge: Cambridge University Press, 2003); Mark Coeckelbergh, *The Metaphysics of Autonomy: The Reconciliation of Ancient and Modern Ideals of the Person* (Basingstoke: Palgrave Macmillan, 2004); John Christman and Joel Anderson, eds., *Autonomy and the Challenges to Liberalism: New Essays* (Cambridge: Cambridge University Press, 2005); Taylor, ed., *Personal Autonomy*; Marina A. L. Oshana, *Personal Autonomy in Society* (Aldershot, England: Ashgate Publishing, 2006); John Davenport, *Will as Commitment and Resolve: An Existential Account of Creativity, Love, Virtue, and Happiness* (New York: Fordham University Press, 2007).

8. Dworkin, *The Theory and Practice of Autonomy*, 31–32; discussed in Donald C. Ainslie, "Bioethics and the Problem of Pluralism," in *Bioethics*, eds. Ellen Frankel Paul, Fred D. Miller Jr., Jeffrey Paul, 9 (Cambridge: Cambridge University Press, 2002). For further discussion of the view that persons who are autonomous with respect to their decisions must value their autonomy, see Chapter 5.

9. For the sake of brevity it will no longer be explicitly noted that the discussion in this volume is concerned only with *Western* bioethics.

10. Frankfurt, "Freedom of the Will and the Concept of a Person," 24–25.

NOTES TO CHAPTER 1

1. Stephen Darwall notes that this is a "commonplace" recognition; see his "The Value of Autonomy and Autonomy of the Will," *Ethics* 116, no. 2 (2006): 263.
2. Gertrude Stein was here referring to Oakland, where she spent her childhood. Gertrude Stein, *Everybody's Autobiography* (New York: Cooper Square Publishers, 1971), 289.
3. Harry Yeide Jr., "The Many Faces of Autonomy," *Journal of Clinical Ethics* 3, no. 4 (1992): 269–274; Susan J. Dwyer, "The Many Faces of Autonomy," *The Philosophers' Magazine* 13 (2001): 40–41; H. Tristram Engelhardt Jr., "The Many Faces of Autonomy," *Health Care Analysis* 9, no. 3 (2001): 283–297.
4. This is the approach that John Christman adopts; see his "Introduction," in *The Inner Citadel: Essays on Individual Autonomy*, ed. Christman, 4–5 (New York: Oxford University Press, 1989).
5. See, for example, Joel Feinberg, "Autonomy," in *The Inner Citadel*, ed. Christman, 28, and Marina A. L. Oshana, "Wanton Responsibility," *The Journal of Ethics* 2, no. 1 (1998): 262; *Personal Autonomy in Society*, 77.
6. See, respectively, Richard Double, "Two Types of Autonomy Accounts," *Canadian Journal of Philosophy* 22, no. 1 (1992): 65–80; Christman, "Introduction," 6–12; Laura Waddell Ekstrom, "A Coherence Theory of Autonomy," *Philosophy and Phenomenological Research* 53, no. 3 (1993): 599–616; Harry G. Frankfurt, "Coercion and Moral Responsibility," in *The Importance of What We Care About*, ed. Frankfurt, 42–43 (Cambridge: Cambridge University Press, 1988). Note that recognizing Frankfurt holds autonomy to be a property of person's actions does not conflict with the claim in Chapter 3 that he does not have an account of what it is for a person to be autonomous with respect to her effective first-order desires. For a related discussion of this distinction between a person's identification with her effective first-order desires and her autonomy with respect to her actions, see James Stacey Taylor, "Autonomy, Duress, and Coercion," *Social Philosophy & Policy* 20, no. 2 (2003): 133–138.
7. If all things are equal with respect to the number of local attributes that a person is autonomous with respect to, a person will possess a greater degree of autonomy over her life to the degree that she is autonomous with respect to her local attributes that are of greater import to her. Noting this moves towards capturing the intuition that persons can be autonomous with respect to their lives—a global attribution of autonomy—but it does so in a way that is firmly rooted in considering autonomy to be a property of persons with respect to their local attributes.
8. Generally, but not universally; see Dworkin, *The Theory and Practice of Autonomy*, 21. It seems that, here, Dworkin is confusing a person's being autonomous with respect to her actions with her acting authentically.
9. For further discussion of this see Taylor, "Autonomy, Duress, and Coercion," 127–155.
10. See, for example, John Christman, "Liberalism, Autonomy, and Self-Transformation," *Social Theory and Practice* 27, no. 2 (2001): 201.
11. Paul M. Hughes, "Ambivalence, Autonomy, and Organ Sales," *Southern Journal of Philosophy*, 44, no. 2 (2006): 237–251.
12. See, for example, Dworkin, *The Theory and Practice of Autonomy*, 16.
13. William Shakespeare, *Othello*, ed. Edward Pechter (New York: W. W. Norton & Company, 2003).
14. This example will be discussed further in Chapters 3, 8, and 9.

15. Alfred R. Mele, *Autonomous Agents: From Self-Control to Autonomy* (New York: Oxford University Press) 180, 181.

16. The example of Iago and Othello shows that Michael McKenna is mistaken to assert that Mele is wrong to hold that King George suffers from a diminution in his autonomy when he is subject to the manipulations of his staff. McKenna holds that Mele is mistaken here because King George "can be understood to act in light of rules that . . . [he] . . . accepts as . . . [his] . . . own." (McKenna, "The Relationship Between Autonomous and Morally Responsible Agency," 210–211.) Yet although King George and Othello are acting in light of rules that they accept as their own, their beliefs concerning their circumstances have been manipulated by other persons to ensure that when they act in accordance with these rules they perform the actions that their manipulators have decided that they will perform. As such, then, the examples of King George and Othello show that a person's acting in accordance with rules that she accepts as her own is insufficient to ensure that she is autonomous with respect to her decisions or her actions. See Mele, *Autonomous Agents*, 182.

17. Mele, *Autonomous Agents*, 181.

18. This point was noted by McKenna, "The Relationship Between Autonomous and Morally Responsible Agency," 210.

19. The point of this example—that for a person to suffer from a loss of control over his decisions, desires, and actions as a result of the actions of other agents they must be intending to usurp control over her decisions, desires, and actions—can also be used to undermine objections to compatibilist accounts of moral responsibility that compare a person who is subject to universal manipulation by other agents (and so is not responsible) to a person whose decisions, desires, and actions are identical to those of the manipulated person, but where they are the result of nonintentional forces beyond his control. For an example of such an objection, see Robert Kane, *Free Will and Values* (Albany, NY: State University of New York Press, 1985), 37–42.

20. Sarah Buss has persuasively argued that "One person can manipulate and deceive another . . .without preventing the manipulated person from governing herself." Sarah Buss, "Valuing Autonomy and Respecting Persons: Manipulation, Seduction, and the Basis of Moral Constraints," *Ethics* 113, no. 2 (2005): 197. Although on the face of it this seems to undermine the above claim that Othello suffered from a diminution in his autonomy with respect to his actions when he was subject to the successful manipulations of Iago, this is not the case. Even though Othello was less autonomous with respect to his manipulated decisions and consequent actions as Iago, and not he, was the font of them, Othello was still governing himself in that he was still acting on desires that he wished to have, and wished to move him to act. That is, Othello was still governing himself in the sense of being moved to act by desires that he *identified* with, even though owing to their genesis he was not autonomous with respect to them. This distinction between autonomy and identification will be elaborated in Chapter 3.

21. Or at least, King George would not fail to direct his own decisions and actions because he was under the control of another; it is still possible that he failed to satisfy the other conditions for him to be autonomous with respect to his decisions and actions that will be outlined next.

22. Note that that a person is autonomous with respect to her decision does not mean that she is therefore autonomous with respect to the actions that she performs as a result of it. For a discussion of this point (albeit in the context of a person's being autonomous with respect to her effective first-order desires and her actions) see Taylor, "Autonomy, Duress, and Coercion," 133–138. Note, too, that in that paper a person's identifying with her effective

first-order desire is mistakenly assimilated to her being autonomous with respect to it—although this mistake does not undermine the salience of that discussion for the point made here.

23. If a person is subject to such unsuccessful manipulation she might still suffer from a diminution in the instrumental value of her autonomy as her decisions would typically be made on the basis of false information. (This would not, however, be the case were the would-be manipulator has a mistaken view of the situation at hand, and in trying to manipulate his victim behaved in such a way that the information that she received is *more* accurate than that which she would have received absent his machinations.) Thus, although such unsuccessful manipulation would not adversely affect her autonomy per se, it would still not be blameless from the point of view of a defender of autonomy.

24. It might be tempting to add at this point a counterfactual condition, such that a person's autonomy with respect to her decisions would be diminished to the degree that the decisions that she makes as a result of being subject to manipulation differ from those that she would have made had she been free from this. But this temptation should be resisted, for the degree to which her manipulated decisions differ from those that she would have made were she to be free from manipulation is irrelevant to the question of the degree to which she is subject to the control of another agent. Instead, the question of the degree to which her manipulated decisions differ from those that she would have made were she to be free from manipulation is relevant only to the question of the degree to which such manipulation is likely adversely to affect her well-being.

25. This account of satisfaction is similar to that offered by Frankfurt, in Harry G. Frankfurt, "The Faintest Passion," in *Necessity, Volition, and Love*, ed. Frankfurt, 105 (Cambridge: Cambridge University Press, 1999).

26. This point is discussed further in Chapter 5 in the context of criticizing Natalie Stoljar's criticisms of content-neutral accounts of autonomy, and in Chapter 7 in the context of criticizing extreme voluntarism.

27. For the advantages of this, see Robert Noggle, "The Public Conception of Autonomy and Critical Self-Reflection," *Southern Journal of Philosophy* 35, no. 4 (1997): 507–509.

28. In Double's terms, a person's decision must exemplify her "individual management style" for her to be autonomous with respect to it. See Double, "Two Types of Autonomy Accounts," 68–69.

29. Evelyn Waugh, *Decline and Fall* (London: Chapman Hall, 1974), 45.

30. Frankfurt, "Freedom of the Will and the Concept of a Person," 17.

31. Ibid., 17.

32. Waugh, *Decline and Fall*, 37.

33. See, for example, Tom L. Beauchamp, "Who Deserves Autonomy, and Whose Autonomy Deserves Respect?" in *Personal Autonomy*, ed. Taylor, 319, and Oshana, *Personal Autonomy in Society*, 23.

34. Frankfurt, "Freedom of the Will," 16–18.

35. Moreover, to accept that by definition wantons cannot be autonomous would be to beg the question against this account of autonomy.

36. See Noggle, "The Public Conception of Autonomy and Critical Self-Reflection," 507–509. See also Gerald Dworkin, *The Theory and Practice of Autonomy*, 17.

37. For an explanation of why the ascription of autonomy to a person with respect to her actions on the basis of ascribing autonomy to her with respect to those of her effective first-order desires that led her to perform the acts in question is only a prima facie ascription, see Taylor, "Autonomy, Duress, and Coercion," 133–138.

38. The possibility of such a tripartite taxonomy of desires was first outlined in James Stacey Taylor, "Review of *Necessity, Volition, and Love* by Harry G. Frankfurt," *Philosophical Quarterly* 51, no. 202 (2001): 114–116. Note that desires that are authentically an agent's own but which she is heteronomous with respect to need not be agential desires of the sort discussed in Chapters 3 and 4; they could be desires that are peculiar to her but which she does not have as a result of making decisions in accordance with a decision-making procedure that she is satisfied with.

39. For an account of autonomy as nonalienation see John Christman, "Autonomy and Personal History," *Canadian Journal of Philosophy* 21, no. 1 (1991): 1–24. For a criticism of such views see Michael Bratman, "Identification, Decision, and Treating as a Reason," *Philosophical Topics* 24, no. 2 (1996), 9.

40. The characterization of a nonalienation account of autonomy being one on which an agent is held to be autonomous with respect to (e.g.) her desires if she does not "disown" them is offered by Paul Benson, "Taking Ownership: Authority and Voice in Autonomous Agency," in *Autonomy and the Challenges to Liberalism: New Essays*, eds. John Christman and Joel Anderson, 104 (Cambridge: Cambridge University Press, 2005).

41. John Christman, "Defending Historical Autonomy: A Reply to Professor Mele," *Canadian Journal of Philosophy* 23, no. 2 (1993): 288. See also Christman, "Autonomy and Personal History," 11.

42. Christman added this fourth condition to his account of what it is for an agent to be autonomous with respect to a desire in "Defending Historical Autonomy," 288, in response to objections from Alfred R. Mele, "History and Personal Autonomy," *Canadian Journal of Philosophy* 23, no. 2 (1993): 271–280.

43. Further criticisms of Christman's account of autonomy are outlined in James Stacey Taylor, "Introduction," 10–13.

44. These accounts of what is involved in a person being alienated from her pro-attitudes are offered by John Christman, "Autonomy, Self-Knowledge, and Liberal Legitimacy," in *Autonomy and the Challenges to Liberalism*, eds. Christman and Anderson, 335.

45. Frankfurt's original account of identification is often (mistakenly, as it is not an account of autonomy) taken to be such an account; see Oshana, *Personal Autonomy in Society*, 21–26. The account of autonomy that Ekstrom has developed, however, certainly is. See Ekstrom, "A Coherence Theory of Autonomy," 599–616. Ahistorical accounts of autonomy are vulnerable to this Problem insofar as a third party (such as a horrible hypnotist or a nefarious neurosurgeon) could inculcate into a person a desire together with the appropriate structural relationships that the proponents of the ahistorical theory of autonomy in question hold are sufficient for the person who possesses the desire in question to be autonomous with respect to it. However, since it appears that such invasively inculcated effective first-order desires are paradigmatically alien to their possessors, since the proponents of ahistorical accounts of autonomy seem committed to holding that their possessors are autonomous with respect to them such inculcated desires appear to be counterexamples to their accounts. The Problem of Manipulation is discussed in Taylor, "Introduction," 5–6, and Tomis Kapitan, "Autonomy and Manipulated Freedom," *Philosophical Perspectives* 14 (2000): 81–103. For a discussion of a similar point in the context of analyzing the concept of identification, see Chapter 4.

46. J. David Velleman, "What Happens When Someone Acts?" *Mind* 101, no. 403 (1992): 464–465.

47. Nomy Arpaly, *Unprincipled Virtue: An Inquiry Into Moral Agency* (New York: Oxford University Press, 2003), 5.
48. See, for example, Merle Spriggs, "Can We Help Addicts Become More Autonomous? Inside the Mind of an Addict," *Bioethics* 17, nos. 5–6 (2003): 542–554; Kapitan, "Autonomy and Manipulated Freedom," 84; and Oshana, *Personal Autonomy in Society*, 24–25.
49. It is, as will be argued in Chapter 3, a separate question of whether he took it freely and of his own free will.
50. Frankfurt characterizes such situations as being situations of "Type A." Harry G. Frankfurt, "Three Concepts of Free Action," in *The Importance of What We Care About*, ed. Frankfurt, 47 (Cambridge: Cambridge University Press, 1988).
51. Similar remarks could also be made with respect to persons who are successfully coerced into performing actions that they would not have otherwise performed; such persons will, like persons in Type A situations, still be fully autonomous with respect to both their decisions to accede to the demands of their coercers and their consequent effective first-order desires.

## NOTES TO CHAPTER 2

1. This is good news for the proponents of the second response to the Gertrude Stein Problem adopted in the previous chapter, for it reinforces the view that there is simply not "too many diverse conceptions of autonomy" for their account of autonomy to be a capturing one. Carol Rovane, *The Bounds of Agency* (Princeton, NJ: Princeton University Press, 2007), 236.
2. The five conceptions of autonomy that Rainer Frost develops, for example, fail to capture any of the connotative contours of autonomy, for these are conceptions of autonomy " . . . that persons as citizens of a law-governed political community must reciprocally and generally grant and guarantee each other." "Political Liberty: Integrating Five Conceptions of Autonomy," in *Autonomy and the Challenges to Liberalism*, eds. Christman and Anderson, 229. These conceptions of autonomy (moral, ethical, legal, political, and social autonomy) have thus been developed to provide an account of political liberty within a certain political framework and not to capture the connotative contours of personal autonomy, as these are generally understood.
3. Joel Feinberg, "Autonomy," in *The Inner Citadel*, ed. Christman, 28.
4. Ibid., 28–49.
5. Dworkin, *The Theory and Practice of Autonomy*, 6.
6. Manuel Vargas, "Review of *Personal Autonomy*," ed. James Stacey Taylor, *Notre Dame Philosophical Reviews* (15th August 2006). Online at: http://ndpr.nd.edu/review.cfm?id=7363. Last accessed October 14th, 2008.
7. Arpaly, *Unprincipled Virtue*, 118–125.
8. It is, of course, no objection to the methodology of this chapter that some of the counterexamples presented within it might be based on unusual cases. As Mill noted, one should not object to an argument's (or a conception's) being "pushed to an extreme," for "unless the reasons are good for an extreme case, they are not good for any case." J. S. Mill, *On Liberty*, ed. Elizabeth Rapaport (Indianapolis: Hackett Publishing Company, Inc., 1978), 20.
9. Feinberg, "Autonomy," 43.
10. Christman, "Introduction," 5.
11. Isaiah Berlin, *Four Essays on Liberty*, reprint (Oxford: Oxford University Press, 1969/1977), 122. It should be noted that Berlin's account of the distinction between positive and negative liberty is adopted for exegetical rather

than philosophical reasons, for it is his account of this distinction that Dworkin explicitly adopts in his discussion of the many faces of autonomy.

12. Dworkin cites Joseph Goldstein ("On Being Adult and Being an Adult in Secular Law," in *Adulthood*, ed. E. H. Erikson, 252 [New York: W. W. Norton and Company, 1978]), as equating autonomy with the possession of either negative or positive liberty. (See Dworkin, *The Theory and Practice of Autonomy*, 6.) However, it is not clear that Goldstein is using "autonomy" as synonymous with either negative or positive liberty. As quoted by Dworkin, Goldstein writes "[T]he law is thus implementing its basic commitment to man's autonomy, his freedom to and his freedom from, acknowledge(s) how complex man is." But this quotation could be understood as a list of properties, rather than autonomy being characterized as "freedom to" and "freedom from." Despite this, however, it is clear that Jennifer Jackson, at least, believes that autonomy can be understood as negative liberty, as "autonomy as liberty," in her phrase, for she holds that "In one sense, being autonomous is equivalent to being free—not, for example, constrained by others." Jackson, *Ethics in Medicine* (Cambridge: Polity Press, 2006), 66. This view of autonomy is also endorsed by Bruce Miller, "Autonomy and the Refusal of Lifesaving Treatment," *Hastings Center Report* 11, no. 4 (1981): 22–28. (Miller also discusses autonomy as authenticity, autonomy as effective deliberation—a variety of the understanding of autonomy as reasons-responsiveness that is discussed next—and the Kantian understanding of autonomy as moral reflection.) These understandings of autonomy are discussed as though they were understandings of personal autonomy by Yeide Jr., "The Many Faces of Autonomy," 269–274. But although this understanding of autonomy can be found in the wild (albeit rarely), it is clearly not the understanding of autonomy that is used by autonomy theorists or persons who are familiar with their work, for even wantons might possess negative liberty.

13. Berlin, *Four Essays on Liberty*, 131. That autonomy is understood in this way is noted by Mark Coeckelbergh, *The Metaphysics of Autonomy*, 5.

14. Dworkin, *The Theory and Practice of Autonomy*, 6.

15. Michael McKenna, for example, argues that autonomous agency and morally responsible agency are distinct types of agency; see his "The Relationship Between Autonomous and Morally Responsible Agency," 205–234. In a related vein Marina A. L. Oshana argues that certain (nonautonomous) wantons are responsible agents. See her "Wanton Responsibility," 261–276.

16. Unfortunately, Dworkin offers no textual support for his claims. He cites the work of Joseph Goldstein, Thomas Scanlon, R. P. Wolff, R. S. Peters, Joel Feinberg, R. S. Downie and Elizabeth Tefler, R. F. Dearden, John Rawls, and J. L. Lucas (*The Theory and Practice of Autonomy*, 5–6). The problem that exists with his use of Goldstein's work has already been noted. Of the remaining authors, Wolff, Peters, and Rawls are explicit in the passages Dworkin quotes that they are drawing on a *Kantian* conception of autonomy, not the conception of personal autonomy that is the focus of this volume, and that is also the focus of Dworkin's. Wolff writes that "As Kant argued . . . " prior to offering his characterization of "the autonomous man," Peters writes of " . . . the Kantian conception of autonomy . . .," while Rawls writes that "Kantian constructivism. . . is. . .a procedure of construction in which rationally autonomous agents subject to reasonable constraints agree to public principles of justice." See, respectively, Wolff, *In Defense of Anarchism* (New York: Harper and Row, 1970), 14; Peters, "Freedom and the Development of the Free Man," in *Educational Judgments: Papers in the Philosophy of Education*, ed. James F. Doyle, 130 (London: Routledge, 1973); and Rawls, "Kantian Constructivism in Moral Theory," *The Journal of Philosophy* 77, no.

9 (1980): 554. Downie and Tefler also have a Kantian conception of autonomy insofar as they hold that autonomy is partly constituted by persons' moral individuality. See R. S. Downie and Elizabeth Tefler, "Autonomy," *Philosophy* 15 (1971): 301. Quoted in Dworkin, *The Theory and Practice of Autonomy*, 6. The remaining authors are Scanlon, who holds that "To regard himself as autonomous in the sense I have in mind, a person must see himself as sovereign in deciding what to believe and in weighing competing reasons for action," (Thomas Scanlon, "A Theory of Freedom of Expression," *Philosophy and Public Affairs* 1, no. 2 [1972]: 215); Feinberg, who writes that "I am autonomous if I rule me, and no one else rules I," (Joel Feinberg, "The Idea of a Free Man," in *Educational Judgments*, ed. Doyle, 161); Dearden, who holds that "A person is 'autonomous' to the degree that what he thinks and does cannot be explained without reference to his own activity of mind," (R.F. Dearden, "Autonomy and Education," in *Education and the Development of Reason*, eds. R. F. Dearden, P. H. Hirst, and R. S. Peters, 453 [London: Routledge and Kegan Paul, 1972]); and Lucas, who writes, "I, and I alone, am ultimately responsible for the decisions that I make, and am in that sense autonomous" (J. L. Lucas, *The Principles of Politics* [Oxford: Oxford University Press, 1966], 101.) (All quoted in Dworkin, *The Theory and Practice of Autonomy*, 5–6. Dworkin erroneously attributes the papers by Peters and Feinberg to the volume edited by Dearden et al.) Two points are worth making here. First, read as it stands Dearden's account of autonomy is exceptionally weak, for it is not clear that any agent's thoughts and actions could be explained without reference to their own minds. As such, on its most charitable reading this should be taken as almost a trivially true necessary condition for autonomy, rather than of an account of this concept in its own right. Second, a similar point could be made with respect to all the views that are presented here: that they are all exceptionally thin accounts of autonomy, and so, like the concept of "self rule," should best be understood merely as connotative starting points for analysis rather than as analyses in themselves.

17. See, for example, Bruce Waller's use of the term "autonomy" in *The Natural Selection of Autonomy* (Albany, NY: The State University of New York Press, 1998), 8.

18. Contra Vargas, none of the authors in Taylor's *Personal Autonomy* claim this.

19. The views of autonomy as an ideal and as a frequently possessed property will be discussed next, in the section which addresses Arpaly's discussion of heroic autonomy. The views of autonomy as competence and as authority will also be discussed next, in the section that addresses Arpaly's discussion of normative moral autonomy. The only view of autonomy that is mentioned by Vargas that will not be discussed is that of ownership-taking, which, like the view of autonomy as self-rule, is part of the thin understanding of personal autonomy that is shared by all conceptions of this concept.

20. Arpaly, *Unprincipled Virtue*, 118.

21. Ibid., 118. Although Arpaly does not cite the work of any of these philosophers, their representative accounts of what she terms "agent-autonomy" can be found in the following papers: Frankfurt, "Freedom of the Will and the Concept of a Person," 11–25; Gary Watson, "Free Agency," in *The Inner Citadel*, ed. Christman, 109–122; J. David Velleman, "Identification and Identity," in *Contours of Agency: Essays on Themes from Harry Frankfurt*, eds. Sarah Buss and Lee Overton, 91–123 (Cambridge: MIT Press, 2002); Robert Noggle, "The Public Conception of Autonomy and Critical Self-Reflection,"

496–502; Keith Lehrer, "Reason and Autonomy," in *Autonomy*, eds. Paul, Miller, Paul, 177–198 (Cambridge: Cambridge University Press, 2003).

22. Arpaly, *Unprincipled Virtue*, 118. Note that, and contra Arpaly's implicit claim, it is unlikely that any philosopher working on or with the concept of autonomy would hold that being autonomous would be a matter of having second-order desires alone; certainly none of the persons she cites would hold this. Most obviously, an agent might have a second-order desire about a desire that was another person's first-order desire, and yet her mere possession of this desire would tell us nothing about whether or not the first agent possessed autonomy in any way at all. This example is taken from Keith Lehrer, *Metamind*, 89, who uses it for a different purpose.

23. As will be argued in Chapter 3, Frankfurt's early work was concerned with developing an account of what it is for a person to act freely and of his own free will. This account is aimed at determining when a person's desires are "legitimately attributable to him as his own." (Harry G. Frankfurt, "Reply to Michael E. Bratman," in *Contours of Agency*, eds. Buss and Overton, 88.) Watson aims to show that "the difference between free and unfree actions. . .has nothing at all to do with the truth or falsity of determinism"—a metaphysical project that is akin to Frankfurt's aim of offering an account of what it is for a person to act freely and of her own free will. Lehrer's project is within the ambit of this metaphysical discussion too, for he is concerned to develop an account of what he terms "autonomy" that will "provide us with the dignity of being causal agents in the causal order" (Lehrer, "Reason and Autonomy," 198). These projects stand in contrast with the approaches of Bratman and Noggle, who instead of offering such a descriptive account of the status of a person's desires are attempting to offer a normatively laden account, such that if a person's desire is considered to be her own then they have a claim to play a particular role in her practical reasoning. (For a recognition of this see Frankfurt, "Reply to Michael E. Bratman," 86; see also Noggle, "The Public Conception of Autonomy and Critical Self-Reflection," 496.) Finally, Velleman's project is different still—to provide an account of what it is for a person to identify with a motivational state as his own that is not based on the view that such identification will include that state "into something called the self," but, instead, on the view that a person's identification with certain of his motivational states rests simply "on his capacity to reflect on aspects of his personality and to feel a special relation to some of them." (Velleman, "Identification and Identity," 115.)

24. Arpaly is thus mistaken to take accounts of so-called agent-autonomy to be the lodestone of autonomy accounts—although, of course, as will be noted in Chapter 3 this is a widespread mistake.

25. Although Arpaly does not cite anyone who uses the term "autonomy" in this way, this use of the term appears in Bobbie Farsides, "Consent and the Capable Adult Patient—An Ethical Perspective: Consent and Patient Autonomy," in *Nursing Law and Ethics*, second edition, eds. John Tingle and Alan Cribb, 123 (Oxford: Blackwell, 2002).

26. Arpaly, *Unprincipled Virtue*, 119.

27. Ibid., 119. One might think that the proponents of this view of autonomy would include persons who believe that to be autonomous one might have access to an adequate range of options. See, for example, Joseph Raz, *The Morality of Freedom* (Oxford: Oxford University Press, 1986), 204. Yet this is not the case, for the having of options is not the same as being independent of others. Persons would be autonomous on an options-based view of autonomy under appropriate welfare arrangements that afforded them enough appropriate options—but to have these options they would be dependent

on others and so would not satisfy the condition that is required for them to possess autonomy as personal efficacy. One possible proponent of this view of autonomy is Loren Lomasky, who, in "Autonomy and Automobility," *The Independent Review* 2, no. 1 (1997): 5–28, at times holds the view that insofar as motorists exhibit self-direction driving enhances autonomy.

28. For a discussion of this point, see Marilyn Friedman, "Autonomy and Male Dominance," in *Autonomy and the Challenges to Liberalism*, eds. Christman and Anderson, 150–173 (Cambridge: Cambridge University Press, 2005).

29. Jerome Bixby, "It's a *Good* Life," in *Star of Stars*, ed. Frederik Pohl, 219–240 (Garden City, NY: Doubleday, 1960).

30. Arpaly, *Unprincipled Virtue*, 118. Given this, it is not entirely clear what Arpaly's aim in outlining these various understandings and connotations of "autonomy" is.

31. Ibid., 120. The quotation is from Thomas E. Hill Jr., *Dignity and Practical Reason in Kant's Moral Theory* (Ithaca, NY: Cornell University Press, 1992), 78.

32. Arpaly is right to note that a person who possesses agent-autonomy in Frankfurt's sense need not possess independence of mind. She is thus also right to note that feminists who claim that women should be aided in developing their autonomy, or who criticize Frankfurt's analysis of so-called agent-autonomy for failing to explain why a deferential woman suffers from a lack of autonomy, are equivocating without recognizing this. It should be noted, however, that not all criticisms of autonomy that are made from a feminist perspective are based on this error. Carol Gilligan, for example, criticizes Kohlberg's account of autonomy for reflecting a masculine bias on the grounds that it requires that autonomous agents make decisions from an impersonal point of view rather than from the feelings that arise from their personal relationships. Whatever the merits of this criticism, it is clear that it does not stem from misconstruing so-called agent-autonomy to be an account of personal autonomy. See Carol Gilligan, *In a Different Voice* (Cambridge: Harvard University Press, 1982), and Lawrence Kohlberg, "Stage and Sequence: the Cognitive Development Approach to Socialization," in *The Handbook of Social Theory and Research*, ed. D. A. Goslin, 347–480 (Chicago: Rand McNally, 1969). This debate is discussed in Hill, *Dignity and Practical Reason*, 78. Bernard Berofsky claims that an autonomous person must possess personal efficacy as a character trait. See his *Liberation from Self*, 43.

33. The following discussion of Arpaly's account of autonomy as normative moral competence can apply *mutatis mutandis* to Vargas's account of autonomy as competence for medical decision-making.

34. Arpaly, *Unprincipled Virtue*, 120.

35. Ibid., 121.

36. Ibid., 120.

37. Ibid., 120–121.

38. Ibid., 121.

39. It is not clear that in failing to respect his victim's autonomy the thief has thereby violated it, as Arpaly claims—but since nothing hangs on this distinction in this discussion this can be allowed to pass.

40. Assume here that he did not engage in any form of privacy-violating stalking behavior prior to kidnapping them; for further discussion of the relationship between privacy and autonomy and an argument for the view that Clegg could have compromised the autonomy of his victims prior to kidnapping them by stalking them, see Chapter 8.

41. Arpaly, *Unprincipled Virtue*, 120.

42. It should be noted that this argument in favor of Arpaly's view that normative moral autonomy is distinct from agent-autonomy is a better one than that which Arpaly herself develops. Arpaly holds that agent-autonomy must be distinct from normative moral autonomy on the grounds that the latter's commitment to holding that a person who made a decision based on incomplete or misleading data would thereby suffer from compromised autonomy would make autonomy rare, and that since the proponents of agent-autonomy do not believe that it is these conceptions of autonomy must be distinct. (Note again that this is a mischaracterization of the views of the proponents of normative moral autonomy.) However, Arpaly need not invoke any considerations concerning the scarcity or otherwise of autonomy, for she could simply note that, unlike the proponents of normative moral autonomy, for the proponents of agent-autonomy the quality of the data that a person makes his or her decisions upon is simply irrelevant to the question of whether she enjoys agent-autonomy (i.e., identifies with) with her effective first-order desires. And this is a much more straightforward argument for this distinction than that which Arpaly herself makes—although, as was argued previously, it will provide only cold comfort to her with respect to her overall end of trying to show that there are many different senses of autonomy, for (as will be argued in Chapter 3) agent-autonomy is not a conception of autonomy as this concept is commonly understood.

43. In fairness to Arpaly it should be noted that if her claim is simply that normative moral autonomy (i.e., that account of autonomy on which a person's autonomy is compromised by his being subject to deception) is distinct from agent-autonomy (i.e., identification) then she will be correct to hold that normative moral autonomy and agent-identification are distinct—indeed, showing this will be the aim of Chapter 3. However, it seems that Arpaly does not wish to hold that agent-autonomy is not a form of autonomy at all (indeed, in holding that it is "the sense of 'autonomy' that autonomous-action theorists are looking for" she places it at the core of the discussion of autonomy), and, moreover, that she wishes to hold both that normative moral autonomy is simply one further account of autonomy among many, and that (and relatedly) it is a relatively marginal one in the philosophical discussion of autonomy (insofar as it is not that which "autonomous-action theorists" are looking for).

44. See Chapter 3.

45. Harry G. Frankfurt, "Autonomy, Necessity, and Love," in Frankfurt, ed., *Necessity, Volition, and Love*, 132.

46. Velleman, "Identification and Identity," 92.

47. Ibid., 132.

48. Harry G. Frankfurt, "The Importance of What We Care About," in *The Importance of What We Care About*, ed. Frankfurt, 86 (Cambridge: Cambridge University Press, 1988).

49. Ibid., 87.

50. Harry G. Frankfurt, "Rationality and the Unthinkable," in *The Importance of What We Care About*, ed. Frankfurt, 184.

51. Ibid., 183. Arpaly mischaracterizes Frankfurt's example of Lord Fawn and Andy Gowran as one of "a man who decides to spy on his bride-to-be and finds himself forced to stop because the idea of such spying revolts him too much." Arpaly, *Unprincipled Virtue*, 121.

52. Velleman, "Identification and Identity," 97. Velleman denies the claim that there are such motivational essences, but the focus here will be on his criticism that Frankfurt conflates autonomy with authenticity.

53. Ibid., 97. Velleman cites here D. W. Winnicott, "Ego Distortion in Terms of True and False Self," in *The Maturational Processes and the Facilitating*

*Environment*, ed. D. W. Winnicott, 140–152 (London: Hogarth Press, 1965). (Velleman mistakenly cites this article as appearing in D. W. Winnicott, ed., *Collected Papers: Through Pediatrics to Psycho-Analysis* [London: Tavistock Publications, 1958].)

54. Velleman, "Identification and Identity," 97.
55. Ibid., 97. A similar example is offered by Arpaly, *Unprincipled Virtue*, 122.
56. Not only is authenticity not sufficient for autonomy, but it is not necessary, either, as will be argued in Chapter 3. But, as will be argued in Chapter 7, this does not mean that Frankfurt's discussions of volitional necessity and unthinkability are unimportant for discussions of autonomy.
57. See Timothy Schroder and Nomy Arpaly, "Alienation and Externality," *Canadian Journal of Philosophy* 29, no. 3 (1999): 371–388.
58. Arpaly, *Unprincipled Virtue*, 124.
59. Gary Watson, "Free Agency," 112.
60. Arpaly, *Unprincipled Virtue*, 123. For an outline of Frankfurt's usage of these metaphors, see Chapter 3.
61. Arpaly, *Unprincipled Virtue*, 124.
62. Similar remarks also apply to the conception of autonomy as an ideal that Vargas noted.
63. Arpaly, *Unprincipled Virtue*, 125.
64. Arpaly is here referring to so-called agent-autonomy, but her remarks apply equally to personal autonomy.
65. Ibid., 125.
66. Ibid., 51–52.

## NOTES TO CHAPTER 3

1. Frankfurt, "Freedom of the Will and the Concept of a Person," 11–25.
2. Ibid., 20.
3. For a discussion of the role that autonomy is intended to play in discussion of informed consent, see Chapter 10. For a discussion of autonomy in the context of the debate over the morality of markets in human organs, see Taylor, *Stakes and Kidneys*; for an extensive discussion of it in the context of human reproduction see Carolyn McLeod, *Self-Trust and Reproductive Autonomy* (Cambridge: MIT Press, 2002).
4. Frankfurt, "Freedom of the Will and the Concept of a Person," 24. Note that, for Frankfurt, a person might act freely and of his own free will and yet not possess freedom of the will.
5. For an initial discussion of this point see James Stacey Taylor, "Autonomy and Political Liberalism," *Social Theory and Practice* 32, no. 3 (2006): 501–506, and James Stacey Taylor, "Autonomy, Inducements, and Organ Sales," in *Philosophical Reflections on Medical Ethics*, ed. Nafsika Athanassoulis, 137–140 (London: Palgrave Macmillan, 2005).
6. John Christman and Joel Anderson recognize that "Frankfurt's view is not explicitly an account of autonomy, but rather of freedom of the will." "Introduction," in *Autonomy and the Challenges to Liberalism*, eds. Christman and Anderson, 20, n. 7. For a criticism of their claim that Frankfurt's hierarchical view is an account of what it is for a person to enjoy freedom of the will, rather than of what it is for a person to act freely of his own free will, see Taylor, "Autonomy and Political Liberalism," 503, n. 12.
7. Frankfurt, "Freedom of the Will and the Concept of a Person," 25; Gerald Dworkin, "Autonomy and Behavior Control," *Hastings Center Report* 6, no. 1 (1976), 23.

8. Frankfurt, "Freedom of the Will and the Concept of a Person," 18.
9. Ibid., 25. Note that Frankfurt is using the term "will" here in its Hobbesian sense of "the last Appetite, or Aversion, immediately adhaering [sic] to the action, or to the omission thereof, is that wee [sic] call the WILL . . ." Thomas Hobbes, *Leviathan* (London: Penguin Classics, 1982), pt. I, chap. VI. For a discussion of Frankfurt's differing use of the term "will," see Stefaan Cuypers, "Harry Frankfurt on the Will, Autonomy, and Necessity," *Ethical Perspectives* 5, no. 1 (1998): 44–52.
10. Gerald Dworkin, "Autonomy and Behavior Control," 24.
11. Ibid., 25.
12. See, for example, Taylor, "Introduction," 4; David Shoemaker, "Caring, Identification, and Agency," *Ethics* 114, no. 1 (2003): 88–89; Arpaly, *Unprincipled Virtue*, chap. 4. Perhaps the most influential person in this regard is John Christman, who took Frankfurt to "provide an account of individual autonomy" in "Freedom of the Will and the Concept of a Person." That *The Inner Citadel* (Christman, "Introduction," 7) came to be an extremely influential collection of papers on autonomy no doubt solidified and stimulated the view that Frankfurt and Dworkin provided similar hierarchical analyses of autonomy.
13. This is simply intended to be an outline of the intuitive basis of identification and autonomy, not an account of each concept.
14. Thalberg takes this to indicate a serious weakness in the hierarchical views developed by Frankfurt and Dworkin, for he believes that they can only accommodate this intuition by attributing implausible motivations to the victims of coercion. Irving Thalberg, "Hierarchical Analyses of Unfree Action," in *The Inner Citadel*, ed. Christman, 126. For a response to Thalberg and a more extended discussion of the relationship between identification, autonomy, and coercion, see Taylor, "Autonomy, Duress, and Coercion," 133–138.
15. Although this claim exemplifies a standard—and plausible—understanding of the relationship between addiction and autonomy, it is incorrect.
16. Frankfurt, "Freedom of the Will and the Concept of a Person," 24.
17. Ibid., 24.
18. Ibid., 24.
19. For further discussion of this point, see Taylor, "Autonomy, Inducements, and Organ Sales," 137–140.
20. That this supplementary account differs in important respects from Frankfurt's original account thus does not undermine the claims concerning identification, previously, for they are also applicable to this account of identification.
21. Dworkin, *The Theory and Practice of Autonomy*, 9. Dworkin is here writing of judgmental relevance with respect to autonomy, but his comments are equally applicable to accounts of any concept.
22. The account of identification that will be developed in this volume will thus draw from Frankfurt's account of decisive identification. See Frankfurt, "Identification and Wholeheartedness," in *The Importance of What We Care About*, ed. Frankfurt, 167–174.
23. As noted in the previous chapter and as will be further outlined later, this does not preclude a person's agential desires being *authentically* hers *qua* agent.
24. As outlined in Taylor, "Autonomy, Duress, and Coercion," 152–155, successfully subjecting a person to coercion compromises his autonomy in a different way than successfully subjecting him to either manipulation or deception, although it still achieves this end by affecting the decision that the

person in question makes. This is because, in brief, in successfully coercing a person into performing certain actions a coercer brings it about that his victim decides to relinquish control over his actions to him.

25. For an example of such an objection (here leveled against Frankfurt's early hierarchical analysis of what Christman believed to be autonomy), see Christman, "Autonomy and Personal History," 8. Examples of internalist theories of autonomy against which this type of objection could be effective include Ekstrom, "A Coherence Theory of Autonomy," 599–616; and Lehrer, "Reason and Autonomy," 177–198. Note that although, strictly speaking, a theory of autonomy will be primarily a theory of what makes a person autonomous with respect to her decisions, as was outlined in the Introduction this is a revisionary understanding of autonomy, and so for the sake of exegetical accuracy concerning other accounts of autonomy it is accepted that they focus on what it is for a person to be autonomous with respect to her effective first-order desires.

26. Nomy Arpaly, "Responsibility, Applied Ethics, and Complex Autonomy Theories," in *Personal Autonomy*, ed. Taylor, 165.

27. Ibid., 175.

28. Ibid., 174.

29. Ibid., 174. The previous quotations are from Arpaly's account of the criteria in the *Field Guide*.

30. Ibid., 174. Strangely, Arpaly does not recognize that other complex autonomy theories—such as those offered by Robert Noggle, and Tom L. Beauchamp and James F. Childress—are in accord with the criteria outlined by M. Bauer, *The Field Guide to Psychiatric Assessment and Treatment* (Philadelphia: Lippincott/Williams and Wilkins, 2003). See Noggle, "The Public Conception of Autonomy and Critical Self-Reflection," 495–515, and Tom L. Beauchamp and James F. Childress, *Principles of Biomedical Ethics*, 5th ed. (Oxford: Oxford University Press, 2001), 59–60.

31. Arpaly, "Responsibility, Applied Ethics, and Complex Autonomy Theories," 174.

32. Ibid., 174.

33. It is unclear why Arpaly is suspicious of the importance of autonomy for applied ethics in general. It appears that her criticism of its adoption in areas such as professional ethics, legal ethics, academic ethics, business ethics, and the like is based on a (very hasty) generalization of her points concerning the conditions required for a person to be competent with respect to her medical decisions as outlined in the *Field Guide*, together with her view that such conditions are separate from those that the proponents of complex autonomy theories require to be met for a person to be autonomous with respect to her decisions.

34. There is a further lacuna in Arpaly's argument here, for she rests her case that philosophical discussions of autonomy are removed from the use of this concept in bioethics in particular, and applied ethics in general, on the absence within the *Field Guide* of any philosophically sophisticated account of when a person should be subject to paternalistic intervention. But the fact that a field guide lacks such an account does not show that such an account is lacking in philosophical discussions of medical ethics— it just shows that it is lacking at the level of clinical practice. And this should not surprise us. After all, the mere fact that military training does not include philosophically sophisticated accounts of which persons should legitimately count as combatants does not show that no such accounts are offered, or that they are not useful in practice (e.g., when it comes time to determine who to aim to kill).

35. Arpaly, "Responsibility, Applied Ethics, and Complex Autonomy Theories," 174.
36. Moreover, since a person's identification with his effective first-order desire is not necessary for him to be autonomous with respect to the decision from which it flowed, a person would not need to meet the criteria for identification (such as those Arpaly outlines) for him to be autonomous with respect to his decisions.
37. Paul Benson, "Taking Ownership," 101. In the first set of metaphors Frankfurt is writing of what it is for a person to act freely and of his own free will with no mention of autonomy ("Freedom of the Will and the Concept of a Person," 21, 22). The second set of metaphors refers to a case in which Frankfurt claims that a person's "passivity or impaired autonomy may be due to the force of what is in some basically literal sense the individual's own desires" (Frankfurt, "Identification and Wholeheartedness," 165). However, this does not commit Frankfurt to the view that a person's passivity in the sense of failing to identify with his effective first-order desires is therefore coextensive with his suffering from impaired autonomy, for the "or" in this sentence could be read as treating "passivity" and "impaired autonomy" as distinct impairments, rather than as indicating that they are to be understood as being synonymous.
38. Frankfurt, "Autonomy, Necessity, and Love," in *Necessity, Volition, and Love*, ed. Frankfurt, 133 (Cambridge: Cambridge University Press, 1999).
39. This reason for believing that Frankfurt's work on identification should be understood as being an analysis of autonomy was first offered in Taylor, "Autonomy, Duress, and Coercion," 129, n. 5. Although, as will be argued next, it was mistaken to believe that Frankfurt's terminology offers us any reason to be believe that his account of identification should be understood as an account of autonomy, it should be noted that even this initial argument here came with a caveat: that, for Frankfurt, persons should only be understood as being autonomous with respect to those desires that they reflectively identify with. The reason for this caveat was that in his more recent work on identification Frankfurt held that both persons and nonpersons could identify with their effective first-order desires, with the latter identifying with them without having volitionally endorsed them after reflecting upon them (Frankfurt, "The Faintest Passion," 105–106). Thus, since Frankfurt held that autonomy is grounded in the volitional structure of a person's will ("Autonomy, Necessity, and Love," 132), the type of identification that would be coextensive with autonomy (were any type to be) would be reflective identification. For a further discussion of this latter point see Taylor, "Review of *Necessity, Volition, and Love*," 114–116.
40. Frankfurt, "Autonomy, Necessity, and Love," 130.
41. Ibid., 132. This first aspect of the paper runs from section II to section V, inclusive. That Frankfurt's conception of autonomy as outlined here is similar to the account of what is required for a person to act freely and of his own free will, as outlined previously, does lend support to the view that these concepts are coextensive, for Frankfurt's brief account of autonomy outlined here is also compatible with the account of autonomy that is outlined previously.
42. To defuse the apparent hubris of this claim it should be noted that it is, in the spirit of the title of this chapter, an allusion to Sydney Carton's closing words in Charles Dickens' *A Tale of Two Cities*.

## NOTES TO CHAPTER 4

1. See, for example, Christman, "Introduction," 6–12; Taylor, "Introduction," 18–23; and James Stacey Taylor, "Identification and Quasi-Desires,"

*Philosophical Papers* 34, no. 1 (2005): 111–136. Note that both Christman and Taylor conflate autonomy and identification in these papers.

2. Frankfurt, "Freedom of the Will and the Concept of a Person," 11, n. 1.
3. Ibid., 19.
4. Ibid., 23.
5. Ibid., 16.
6. Ibid., 20. In this context Frankfurt is using the term "will" in its Hobbesian sense, as an effective desire "that moves (or will or would move) a person all the way to action." Ibid., 14.
7. Ibid., 24. For a further discussion of this point see Harry G. Frankfurt, "Alternate Possibilities and Moral Responsibility," in *The Importance of What We Care About*, ed. Frankfurt, 1–10.
8. Frankfurt, "Freedom of the Will and the Concept of a Person," 18.
9. These are outlined in Taylor, "Introduction," 5–10. Note that there Frankfurt's analysis of identification was wrongly held to be an analysis of autonomy.
10. For a discussion of the ontological status of volitions, see Lawrence Haworth, "Dworkin on Autonomy," *Ethics* 102, no. 1 (1991): 130, n. 5.
11. Note that on this version of the Problem of Manipulation the manipulation in question involves the direct implantation of an effective first-order desire and its corresponding volitional endorsement. It does not involve interpersonal manipulation of the sort that Iago subjected Othello to, and nor does it involve merely the inculcation into a person of a desire that he then decides to act on. Noting this is important, for while invasive manipulation of a complete preference structure does appear to serve as a counterexample to Frankfurt's original account of identification, as argued both in this chapter and in Chapter 3 persons subjected to the other two types of manipulation could still identify with the first-order desires that they had a result, even if they could not be said to be autonomous with respect to them.
12. Gary Watson, "Free Agency," 218. Watson's criticism of Frankfurt's initial account of identification could also be understood to be a version of the Ab Initio Problem. See Taylor, "Introduction," 6.
13. Christman, "Introduction," 6–12.
14. Robert Noggle, "Autonomy and the Paradox of Self-Creation: Infinite Regresses, Finite Selves, and the Limits of Authenticity," in *Personal Autonomy*, ed. Taylor, 87.
15. Frankfurt explicitly endorses his view as a compatibilist one; see "Freedom of the Will and the Concept of a Person," 25.
16. Frankfurt recognizes this; see his "Identification and Externality," in *The Importance of What We Care About*, ed. Frankfurt, 65.
17. Note that, as will be argued next, meeting these two conditions is necessary but not sufficient for an account of identification to be satisfactory.
18. For a further discussion of this point see Robert Noggle, "Autonomy, Value, and Conditioned Desire," *American Philisophical Quarterly* 32, no. 1 (1995): 57–69.
19. This account of identification is outlined and defended more fully in Taylor in "Identification and Quasi-Desires," 111–136.
20. On the view outlined here, then, wantons could be persons, for this view does not require that agents assess the desirability of their desires.
21. This has been explicitly recognized by Michael Bratman, who has based his account of identification on a Lockean account of personal identity, and Stefaan E. Cuypers, who has similarly developed an identity-based account of identification. See Michael Bratman, "Planning Agency, Autonomous Agency," in *Personal Autonomy*, ed. Taylor, 42; "Reflection, Planning, and Temporally Extended Agency," in *Structures of Agency: Essays,* ed. Michael

Bratman, 29–31 (New York: Oxford University Press, 2007); "Two Problems About Human Agency," in *Structures of Agency*, ed. Bratman, 99–100; and Cuypers, *Self-Identity and Personal Autonomy*, 85–86.

22. It might be held that this is merely an epistemological problem for the proponents of such a structural approach to analyzing identification, rather than a substantive one. Yet although this is so, without an account of personal identity to undergird such an account it will be incomplete. As such, then, an account of identification that does not require such underpinning is prima facie to be preferred.

23. Frankfurt, "Freedom of the Will and the Concept of a Person," 21.

24. Frankfurt, "Identification and Wholeheartedness," 167.

25. Watson, "Free Agency," 218.

26. Frankfurt, "Identification and Wholeheartedness," 167.

27. Ibid., 167–169.

28. That Frankfurt failed to recognize this is shown by his claim in "The Faintest Passion" that if the final element in a process of identification was "some deliberate psychic element—some deliberate attitude or belief or feeling or intention" that the person in question needed "to think, or to adopt, or to accept," then there would be a danger of a problematic regress since the question could always be raised as to whether the person identified with *that* "psychic element" ("The Faintest Passion," 104). With this claim in hand, Frankfurt developed his account of decisive identification as just outlined to include a satisfaction condition, where to be satisfied with one's higher-order volition (i.e., that which endorses one's effective first-order desire) is a passive state, "a matter of simply *having no interest* in making changes" ("The Faintest Passion," 105). However, since the question of whether or not a person can be alienated from his decisions does not arise as Frankfurt believes it does, there is no need to hold that the final element in a process of identification must be a nondeliberate one. And this is a good thing, for, as Michael Bratman has argued, a person must be active, rather than passive, with respect to his identifications, for otherwise *he* will not be identifying with it at all. See Bratman, "Identification, Decision, and Treating as a Reason," 7.

29. Frankfurt developed these examples for a different purpose.

30. Frankfurt, "Freedom of the Will and the Concept of a Person," 17.

31. Ibid., 24.

32. For further discussion of this see James Stacey Taylor, "Willing Addicts, Unwilling Addicts, and Acting of One's Own Free Will," *Philosophia* 33, nos. 1–4 (2005): 237–262.

33. A person's identifying with a desire is thus not only not sufficient for him to be autonomous with respect to it, as was demonstrated with the example of Iago and Othello in Chapter 3, but it is not necessary for this, either. This is because it is possible for a person to direct himself to act on an agential desire, and thus be autonomous with respect both to it and the actions that it motivates him to perform. A person, then, can be autonomous with respect to a desire with which he does not identify. Any lingering air of paradox concerning this observation should be dispelled by recalling that, as was argued in Chapter 3, identification and autonomy are distinct concepts.

34. Velleman, "What Happens When Someone Acts?" 464.

35. Ibid., 464.

36. A version of this objection has been offered by Christman, "Introduction," 10.

37. Frankfurt, "Identification and Externality," 62.

38. Denise Meyerson, "When Are My Actions Due to Me?" *Analysis* 54, no. 3 (1994): 172. Meyerson here cites David Pears, *Motivated Irrationality*

(Oxford: Clarendon Press, 1984), 204–205, who developed this point for another purpose.

39. For a discussion of a similar point see Oshana, "Wanton Responsibility," 261–276.

40. Such a tripartite taxonomy of desires was first outlined in Taylor, "Review of *Necessity, Volition, and Love*," 114–116.

## NOTES TO CHAPTER 5

1. Sigurdur Kristinsson, "The Limits of Neutrality: Toward a weakly substantive account of autonomy," *Canadian Journal of Philosophy* 30, no. 2 (2000): 266. Kristinsson offers as an example of a procedural account of autonomy that of John Christman, in his "Autonomy and Personal History," and an example of a structural account that of Laura Waddell Ekstrom, "A Coherence Theory of Autonomy." (Kristinsson, "The Limits of Neutrality," 266, n. 17 and n. 18.) He also claims that Frankfurt's account of identification (as exemplified in his papers "Freedom of the Will and the Concept of a Person," "Identification and Wholeheartedness," and "The Faintest Passion"), is a structural account of autonomy, but this is mistaken for the reasons outlined in Chapter 3.

2. This distinction between strongly and weakly substantive accounts of autonomy is outlined in Kristinsson, "The Limits of Neutrality," 258–259. It is not clear, however, that this distinction is a tenable one, for since weakly substantive conceptions of autonomy simply preclude persons from adopting certain evaluative outlooks if they are to be considered autonomous with respect to their actions, a weakly substantive account of autonomy could be transformed into a strongly substantive account simply by requiring that a person possess the converse evaluative attitude of that which it precludes. Moreover, as Paul Benson has argued, to call negative substantive account of autonomy "weakly" substantive and to hold that their cousins that impose positive requirement upon persons' evaluative outlooks "strongly" substantive is misleading, "as negative forms of normative requirement could prove to impose many demanding constraints on autonomous agents, whereas a positive normative requirement might involve nothing more than a single, relatively permissive value." Paul Benson, "Feminist Intuitions and the Normative Substance of Autonomy," in *Personal Autonomy*, ed. Taylor, 139, n. 11.

3. Advocating a framework such as this for bioethical and medical decision-making should not be read as an endorsement of value relativism, but of fallibilism. A devout Christian, for example, could endorse this autonomy-based pluralistic approach to decision-making while still holding that the decisions that persons might make within it (such as the decision to procure an abortion, for example) are utterly immoral. The general political approach that lies behind the advocacy of a decision-making framework such as this would be in the spirit of classical liberalism.

4. This was recognized by Janet Smith in "The Pre-eminence of Autonomy in Bioethics," 182–195.

5. Note that a concern about the imposition of values upon persons who do not share them is not always a concern about healthcare professionals imposing their values upon their patients; it is also a concern about patients imposing (or attempting to impose) their values upon healthcare professionals, by, for example, demanding that they provide them with medical services (such as abortions) or products (such as certain forms of the morning-after pill) that they are morally opposed to.

6. Kristinsson, "The Limits of Neutrality," 257.

7. Dworkin, *The Theory and Practice of Autonomy*, 129; quoted by Kristinsson, "The Limits of Neutrality," 257.

8. John Christman, "Liberalism and Individual Positive Freedom," *Ethics* 101, no. 2 (1991): 359; quoted by Kristinsson, "The Limits of Neutrality," 357–358. It should be noted that although Christman's account of autonomy is undoubtedly a content-neutral one, this quotation does not support the view that it is as clearly as Kristinsson believes. As will be shown below, while this quotation might preclude Christman's account of autonomy from being a normative competence account of autonomy, it does not preclude it from being a substantive account of autonomy.

9. Double, "Two Types of Autonomy Accounts," 65–80.

10. Kristinsson, "The Limits of Neutrality," 259–260.

11. Ibid., 261.

12. Ibid., 266.

13. Ibid., 266.

14. Ibid., 267. Kristinsson cites Christman's papers, "Liberalism and Individual Positive Freedom," "Autonomy and Personal History," and "Defending Historical Autonomy." Christman's account of the conditions that must be met for a person to be autonomous with respect to a desire is quoted and criticized in Chapter 1.

15. Kristinsson, "The Limits of Neutrality," 267. The need to separate the conditions that must be met for a person to be autonomous with respect to her effective first-order desires from those that must be met for her to be autonomous with respect to her actions is discussed more fully in Taylor, "Autonomy, Duress, and Coercion," 127–155.

16. Kristinsson, "The Limits of Neutrality," 268. Kristinsson here cites Jon Elster, "Sour Grapes—Utilitarianism and the Genesis of Wants," in *The Inner Citadel*, ed. Christman, 170–176.

17. Kristinsson, "The Limits of Neutrality," 268.

18. Ibid., 268.

19. Ibid., 269; Kristinsson here cites Dworkin, *The Theory and Practice of Autonomy*, 15–18.

20. Kristinsson, "The Limits of Neutrality," 270; Kristinsson here cites Dworkin, *The Theory and Practice of Autonomy*, 16.

21. Kristinsson, "The Limits of Neutrality," 270.

22. Ibid.

23. Dworkin, "Autonomy and Behavior Control," 24.

24. That Dworkin's views should best be construed this way has been argued for in Taylor, *Stakes and Kidneys*, chap. 2.

25. A person who wished to defend Dworkin's content-neutral account of autonomy along these lines would be defending a hybrid account of autonomy that would stem from his earlier and later accounts. Dworkin's earlier account of autonomy, as outlined in "Autonomy and Behavior Control," was a substantive account, in that it required a person to exhibit "substantive independence" with respect to the formation of his preferences to be autonomous with respect to them. That is, it required that a person's preferences not be influenced by the needs, expectations, or predicaments of others, and so placed value-laden constraints upon which preferences a person could be autonomous with respect to. In Dworkin's later account of autonomy he dropped the requirement that a person exhibit substantive independence but held that autonomy was global property, rather than a punctuate one. Thus, to defend Dwokin's account of autonomy as a content-neutral account in the way outlined previously, one will have to jettison the substantive independence condition from his earlier

account, and jettison the global approach from the later account, to provide an account of autonomy on which a person is autonomous with respect to his preferences if he critically reflects upon them, and endorses them in the light of this critical reflection, and that this critical reflection is performed under conditions of procedural independence (e.g., free from manipulation and deception).

26. Kristinsson, "The Limits of Neutrality," 257.

27. Such open-textured desires are discussed more fully in Taylor, "Autonomy, Duress, and Coercion," 150–155.

28. Kristinsson, "The Limits of Neutrality," 257.

29. It might be objected that conditions that Christman outlines for a person to be autonomous with respect to her pro-attitudes do not require that the person whose autonomy is in question must herself value critical reflection, for they only require that she would not have rejected the pro-attitude in question had she been attending to its development. Since this counterfactual condition can be met without any actual critical reflection taking place, it might, such an objector could urge, be possible on Christman's account of autonomy for a person to be autonomous with respect to her pro-attitudes without herself valuing critical reflection, and so without ever having engaged in this. However, a person's failure to value reflection would violate the second of Christman's conditions for a person to be autonomous with respect to her pro-attitudes: that her lack of resistance to the attitude in question "did not take place (or would not have) under the influence of factors that inhibit self-reflection," for a person's failure to value self-reflection would be such a factor. Christman, "Defending Historical Autonomy," 288.

30. This point could also be made with respect to Elster's account.

31. The sort of reasons that are at issue here will be normatively laden ones, such as those imposed by moral obligations. Noting this is important, for not only is it a descriptively accurate account of the class of reasons that are of concern to persons who offer normative competence theories of autonomy but it also precludes them from being subject to the criticism that it is implausible to hold that a person lacks autonomy just because he is ignorant of certain facts about his situation. (For a development of this point, consider the case of Martin Frobisher discussed in Chapter 1.) As such, John Santiago is mistaken to claim that substantive theorists of autonomy are concerned with the factual content of person's motives. John Santiago, "Personal Autonomy: What's Content Got to Do with It?" *Social Theory and Practice* 31, no. 1 (2005): 80. That Santiago is writing of normative competence theories (although he does not recognize this) is clear when he writes that "in reflecting upon the desire to become a plantation slave owner, a substantive theorist would reject an endorsement of the desire on the basis that *the content of it tracks* neither the reality of the contemporary U.S. economy nor the moral standing of all people." (Santiago, "Personal Autonomy," 79–80; emphasis added).

32. Henry Richardson, "Autonomy's Many Normative Presuppositions," *American Philosophical Quarterly* 38, no. 3 (1991): 287–303. Note that the conclusion of Richardson's argument is much stronger than the conclusion of the argument given, in which it was held that Elster's, Christman's, and Dworkin's analyses of autonomy are *minimally* substantive analyses of autonomy insofar as they require that a person endorse the value of critical reflection to be autonomous with respect to her pro-attitudes, for Richardson believes that the normative presuppositions that undergird the ascription of withholding of the property of autonomy to persons with respect to their actions are considerably more substantive than this.

33. Ibid., 288. Again, note that this claim about value pursuit is considerably stronger than the minimal claims concerning the need for an autonomous person not to cede control over her actions and to value critical reflection.
34. Jon Elster, *Sour Grapes: Studies in the Subversion of Rationality* (Cambridge: Cambridge University Press, 1983).
35. Richardson, "Autonomy's Many Normative Presuppositions," 292.
36. Ibid., 293.
37. Ibid., 294.
38. Ibid., 294.
39. Richard Double, "Two Types of Autonomy Accounts," 77. Quoted by Richardson, "Autonomy's Many Normative Presuppositions," 294.
40. Ibid., 294.
41. For an additional discussion of Richardson's example of the fox and Bully Stryver, see Friedman, "Autonomy and Male Dominance," 160–161.
42. Richardson, "Autonomy's Many Normative Presuppositions," 293.
43. Since these reasons would be factual rather than normative, Richardson is here not drawing on an intuition that would support a normative competence approach to autonomy of the sort that will be discussed next.
44. Ibid., 303, and 294, respectively.
45. Ibid., 303, n. 24.
46. Ibid., 294.
47. Natalie Stoljar, "Autonomy and the Feminist Intuition," in *Relational Autonomy: Feminist Perspectives on Autonomy, Agency, and the Social Self*, eds. Catriona Mackenzie and Natalie Stoljar, 95 (Oxford: Oxford University Press, 2000). Kristin Luker, *Taking Chances: Abortion and the Decision Not to Contracept* (Berkeley, CA: University of California Press, 1975).
48. Stoljar, "Autonomy and the Feminist Intuition," 109. Here Stoljar differs from Irving Thalberg, who claims that women who embrace such norms might lack autonomy as they were manipulated into doing so. (See his "Socialization and Autonomous Behavior," *Tulane Studies in Philosophy* 28 (1979): 27–32.) For Stoljar, it is the content of the norms themselves that precludes the women who embrace them from being autonomous. It should be noted that not all of the women in Lukers's study satisfy the conditions that are required by content-neutral analyses of autonomy; Stoljar notes this, and focuses the "feminist intuition" on those who do.
49. Stoljar, "Autonomy and the Feminist Intuition," 109.
50. Benson, "Feminist Intuitions and the Normative Substance of Autonomy," 131; Diana Tietjens Meyers, "Intersectional Identity and the Authentic Self? Opposites Attract!" in *Relational Autonomy*, eds. Mackenzie and Stoljar, 152. Note that this is not the same point as that made by Flint Schier, discussed in Chapter 6, for Meyers is writing in the content of internalized norms rather than physical constraints.
51. Diana Tietjens Meyers, "Feminism and Womens' Autonomy: The Challenge of Female Genital Cutting," *Metaphilosophy* 31, no. 5 (2000): 475.
52. Benson, "Feminist Intuitions and the Normative Substance of Autonomy," 129.
53. Ibid., 129.
54. The caveat here is required to recognize that a person whose value-set precluded her from exercising reflexive self-awareness would not meet the Degree Condition for autonomy.
55. Benson, "Feminist Intuitions and the Normative Substance of Autonomy," 131.
56. Ibid., 132.
57. Ibid., 132.

58. Oshana, *Personal Autonomy in Society*, 64.
59. Ibid., 64.
60. Santiago, "Personal Autonomy," 84.
61. Ibid., 84.
62. Benson, "Feminist Intuitions and the Normative Substance of Autonomy," 133.
63. Ibid., 133–134.
64. Thomas Hill Jr., "Servility and Self-Respect," in *Autonomy and Self-Respect*, ed. Thomas Hill Jr., 15 (Cambridge: Cambridge University Press, 1991).
65. For an account of such conditions, see Stephen Kershnar, "A Liberal Case for Slavery," *Journal of Social Philosophy* 34, no. 4 (2003): 510–536.
66. John Milton, *Paradise Lost* (London: Penguin Classics, 2000), Book IV.
67. Note that it is not being claimed here that the potential slave would be autonomous once he was enslaved but merely that he could be autonomous with respect to his consent to being enslaved.

## NOTE TO CHAPTER 6

1. See, for example, Thomas Hurka, "Why Value Autonomy?" *Social Theory and Practice* 13, no. 3 (1987): 361–382, and Elisabeth Hildt, "Autonomy and Freedom of Choice in Prenatal Genetic Diagnosis," *Medicine, Health Care and Philosophy* 5, no. 1 (2002): 65–72.
2. See, for example, Gerald Dworkin, "Markets and Morals: The Case for Organ Sales," in *Morality, Harm, and the Law*, ed. Gerald Dworkin, 156 (Boulder, CO: Westview Press, 1994). (Note that Dworkin holds that "markets can increase... autonomy," a claim that, when understood as it is written, is false, for markets do not render persons more autonomous with respect to their decisions and consequent actions. What Dworkin means here, it seems, is that markets can enhance the instrumental value of persons' autonomy to them.) See also Mark J. Cherry, *Kidney for Sale By Owner* (Georgetown: Georgetown University Press, 2005); Taylor, *Stakes and Kidneys*; Amy E. White, "The Morality of an Internet Market in Human Ova," *Journal of Value Inquiry* 40, nos. 2–3 (2006): 311–321.
3. Taylor, *Stakes and Kidneys*, 200.
4. Nafsika Athanassoulis, "Unusual Requests and the Doctor-Patient Relationship," *Journal of Value Inquiry* 40, nos. 2–3 (2006): 259–278.
5. See, for example, Hildt, "Autonomy and Freedom of Choice in Prenatal Genetic Diagnosis," 65–72.
6. Typically, this criticism is offered by persons who wish to argue that certain goods or services should not be market alienable. See, for example, Paul M. Hughes, "Exploitation, Autonomy, and the Case for Organ Sales," *International Journal of Applied Philosophy* 12 no. 1 (1998): 89–95; T. L. Zutlevics, "Markets and the Needy: Organ Sales or Aid?" *Journal of Applied Philosophy* 18, no. 3 (2001): 297–302; and Scott A. Anderson, "Prostitution and Sexual Autonomy: Making Sense of the Prohibition of Prostitution," *Ethics* 112, no. 4 (2002): 748–780.
7. This emphasis is important, for, as will be noted later in this chapter, this conclusion will not have the implications for social policy that the proponents of the view that valuers of autonomy should prefer that persons have fewer choices rather than more often wish their arguments for this view to support.
8. This view is popular among critics of free-market capitalism. See, for example, Joseph Heath, "Liberal Autonomy and Consumer Sovereignty," in

*Autonomy and the Challenges to Liberalism*, eds. Christman and Anderson, 204–225.

9. Indeed, in many cases there are good reasons to reject the conclusions that such discussions of the relationships that hold between autonomy and choices are intended by their authors to support. If so, arguments against them will be briefly noted in the relevant endnotes.

10. It is unlikely that anyone would hold that a person's autonomy would be adversely affected simpliciter simply by the mere appearance of a particular option in her choice-set, irrespective of whether or not she actually chose it. It is, however, plausible to hold that a person's autonomy could be compromised by the presence of certain choices if she chooses to pursue them. If a person chooses to commit suicide, for example, it is clear that her pursuit of this option would (if successful) eliminate her future autonomy.

11. These examples are similar to Arpaly's example (discussed in Chapter 2) of the thief who fails to respect his victim's autonomy by stealing from her but who does not thereby render her less able to exercise her autonomy. It should be recalled, however, that while Arpaly's implicit view of the effect that reducing the number of options that a person has on her autonomy simpliciter is correct, this does not support her contention that there is a distinct type of autonomy that can be termed "normative moral autonomy"—unless (as was noted in Chapter 2) this claim is understood as the claim that autonomy and identification are distinct concepts. (And, as was also noted in Chapter 2, it does not seem that Arpaly intends her claim to be understood in this way.)

12. These are "situations of Type A"; Frankfurt, "Three Concepts of Free Action," 47. The claim that a person who is faced with an unpalatable range of options could still be fully autonomous with respect to the choices that he makes and the actions that he performs in response to them is opposed by Joseph Raz, who maintains that unless persons have an adequate range of options from which to choose they will not be autonomous. Although Raz does not explain how many options, or, more precisely, how many types of options are adequate, he supports his point by reference to two examples: the Man in the Pit and the Hounded Woman. The Man in the Pit's choices are confined to "whether to eat now or a little later, whether to sleep now or a little later, whether to scratch his left ear or not." The Hounded Woman is trapped on a desert island and must expend all of her energy trying to avoid a carnivorous beast (Raz, *The Morality of Freedom*, 374). Despite Raz's claims that neither of these persons are living autonomous lives, it seems more plausible to say that they might be, but that their autonomy is of little instrumental value to them.

13. Hughes, "Exploitation, Autonomy, and the Case for Organ Sales," 89–95.

14. Ibid., 89–95. These uses to which kidney vendors put the money from the sale of their organs are outlined in Madhav Goyal, et al., "Economic and Health Consequences of Selling a Kidney in India," *Journal of the American Medical Association* 288, no. 13 (2002): 1591.

15. Hughes's arguments against allowing persons to sell their nonvital organs are criticized in Taylor, *Stakes and Kidneys*, 75–80.

16. Zutlevics, "Markets and the Needy," 297–302. Zutlevics does not use the term "constraining option" in her argument.

17. Ibid.

18. Zutlevics' argument here is addressed in Taylor, *Stakes and Kidneys*, 80-84.

19. Note that, like Hughes's, Zutlevics's argument is directed at persons who value autonomy instrumentally. There is also another type of option whose presence within the option-set of a population might be beneficial to some but which would adversely affect the majority of the members of the group

in question. Such options might be termed "crowding out options," in that their very presence within the option-set of a group of persons automatically crowds out the existence of other options. Richard Titmuss, in *The Gift Relationship*, argued that the option to sell blood was such an option, in that it would automatically crowd out the option of donating blood in a situation where it could not be sold. As with the argument from group constraining options the argument from crowding out options that is offered to support the claim that a valuer of autonomy should prefer persons to have fewer choices rather than more, is that insofar as such an option would crowd out options that would be attractive to a greater number of persons that the crowding out option itself, a defender of autonomy should advocate precluding such options, for doing so would enable a greater number of persons to exercise their autonomy as they wish. See here Richard Titmuss, *The Gift Relationship: From Human Blood to Social Policy*, ed. Ann Oakley and John Ashton (New York: The New Press, 1997), 307. For a response to Titmuss's argument here see Taylor, *Stakes and Kidneys*, 167–173.

20. The option to plea-bargain is another example of an ultimate constraining option. For an argument to this effect see James Stacey Taylor, "Plea Bargains, Constraining Options, and Respect for Autonomy," *Public Affairs Quarterly* 18, no. 3 (2004): 249–264.

21. Daniel D. Polsby, "Regulation of Foods and Drugs and Libertarian Ideals: Perspectives of a Fellow-Traveller," in *Problems of Market Liberalism*, eds. Ellen Frankel Paul, Fred D. Miller Jr., Jeffrey Paul, 218 (Cambridge: Cambridge University Press, 1998). Polsby cites Henry Blumberg, David Rimland, Donna Carroll, Pamela Terry, and Kaye Wachsmuth, "Rapid Development of Ciprofloxacin Resistance in Methicillin-Susceptable and –Resistant Staphylococcus aureus," *Journal of Infectious Diseases* 163, no. 6 (1991): 1279–1285, among others, in support of this view.

22. Polsby, "Regulation of Foods and Drugs and Libertarian Ideals," 220. Polsby notes that the "Centers for Disease Control in the U.S. have estimated that, for patients infected with antimicrobial-resistant salmonella, hospitalization is necessary more than twice as often as it is for patients who are afflicted with the susceptible strain—57 per cent as compared to 24 per cent." Moreover, Polsby notes, antimicrobial resistant strains of salmonella have over seventeen times the mortality rate of their nonresistant cousins—3.4 per cent compared to 0.2 per cent. Polsby cites Scott Holmberg, Steven Soloman, and Paul Blake, "Health and Economic Impacts of Anti-Microbial Resistance," *Reviews of Infectious Diseases* 9, no. 6 (1987): 1065–1077 as the source of this information.

23. Again, arguments from ultimate constraining options are aimed at persons who value autonomy instrumentally.

24. Restricting the availability of antibiotics need not, however, be the purview of the State, for, as Loren Lomasky has noted (in conversation with Polsby), access to them could also be restricted through extending the property rights that pharmaceutical companies have in them so that they have an incentive to arrange their distribution to guard against their overuse. Noted by Polsby, "Regulation of Foods and Drugs and Libertarian Ideals," 220.

25. For example, R.A. Sells writes that since "the financial benefits [of selling a kidney] [would] have such an impact on the life of the donor. . .as to be irresistible: the element of voluntariness. . .must be. . .in extreme cases, abolished." "Voluntarism of Consent," in *Organ Replacement Therapy: Ethics, Justice, Commerce*, eds. W. Land and J. Dossestor, 20 (New York: Springer-Verlag, 1991). Sells's argument is criticized in Taylor, *Stakes and Kidneys*, 67–69.

26. The first of these arguments from irresistibility can be understood to be directed at persons who believe that autonomy is of intrinsic value. It is, however, not clear whether the second type of argument from irresistibility is aimed at persons who value autonomy intrinsically or instrumentally, for, as will become clear next, this argument is based upon a confused understanding of autonomy.

27. This example of an irresistible offer is taken from Cherry, *Kidney for Sale by Owner*, 92.

28. Note that the adherents of this view are not committed to the view that the more options a person has the more able he is to exercise his autonomy (although some of them might endorse this). Nor are they committed to the view that a person must have a range of options available to her (although, again, some of them might endorse this). Instead, they are only committed to the weaker view that she must believe that she has a range of options open to her.

29. For a discussion of this point see Alan Wertheimer, *Coercion* (Princeton, NJ: Princeton University Press, 1987), 194.

30. Indeed, if the course of action that a person should take is clear to him, owing either to the unthinkability of the alternatives, or to this course of action being required by his volitional nature, then it is plausible to claim that the person concerned will exercise his autonomy *most* fully when he pursues it. See here Frankfurt, "Autonomy, Necessity, and Love," 129–141.

31. See Hughes, "Ambivalence, Autonomy, and Organ Sales," 237–251; Ruth Grant and Jeremy Sugarman, "Ethics in Human Subjects Research: Do Incentives Matter?" *Journal of Medicine and Philosophy* 29, no. 6 (2004): 717–738. This type of argument has been mistakenly characterized as an argument from irresistibility; see Taylor, "Autonomy, Inducements, and Organ Sales," 142–143. This is mistaken, though, since the point of this type of argument is that the desire for the tempting object is not irresistible, and it generates equally strong pro and con attitudes towards it, which leads to the person who is so tempted to suffer from paralyzing motivational ambivalence.

32. The claim here is not that the value of autonomy is purely instrumental; the exercise of autonomy could also be valued for its own sake, insofar as a person could desire to choose for himself for the sake of choosing, even though he realizes that this might be an ineffective way for him to realize his goals. See Claudia Mills, "Choice and Circumstance," *Ethics* 109, no. 1 (1998): 160.

33. Dworkin, *The Theory and Practice of Autonomy*, 80.

34. Flint Schier, "The Kantian Gulag: Autonomy and the Liberal Conception of Freedom," in *Virtue and Taste: Essays on Politics, Ethics, and Aesthetics in Memory of Flint Schier*, eds. Dudley Knowles and John Skorupski, 1–17 (Oxford: Blackwell, 1993). Note that the form of temptation that such persons would be faced with would not be of the sort that would paralyze them, as would the ambivalence-inducing temptation discussed previously.

35. It should be noted that neither Dworkin's argument, nor the response to the Silencing Argument from Irresistibility, show that a person whose first choice would be choice A would necessarily prefer an option-set with only A in it, to an option-set that consists of A together with other (less appealing) options A, B, and C. This is because, first, the having of these options might be desirable to P for reasons unrelated to the exercise of his autonomy. A job candidate who has been offered her dream job might still prefer to have been offered that job together with several others, because she would derive pleasure from being so much in demand. Alternatively, a person might prefer the option-set that includes B and C as well as A because she would enjoy choosing between

the options presented to her, or because if she chose A, rather than merely (albeit happily) accepting it as her only choice she would, post-choice, feel more "ownership" of those aspects of her life that are affected by it.

## NOTES TO CHAPTER 7

1. In both cases a person's decisions will be subject to the constraints of reasons, even though in neither case need she believe that there is an objectively "right" answer concerning what she should do. Holding that there is no objectively right answer concerning what a person should do (including morally) thus does not automatically lead to any form of relativism. For related discussions of this point in the context of bioethical decision-making, see H. Tristram Engelhardt, *The Foundations of Bioethics*, 2nd ed. (New York: Oxford University Press, 1995), and Mark J. Cherry, "Medical Innovation, Collapsing Goods, and the Moral Centrality of the Free Market," *Journal of Value Inquiry* 40, nos. 2–3 (2006): 209–226.
2. Frankfurt, "On the Necessity of Ideals," in *Necessity, Volition, and Love*, ed. Frankfurt, 109. Frankfurt here is writing of what Stefaan E. Cuypers has termed the "substantial will"; see Cuypers, "Harry Frankfurt on the Will, Autonomy, and Necessity," 45.
3. A similar argument is offered by Frankfurt, "On the Necessity of Ideals," 109–111, 114. See also Frankfurt, "Rationality and the Unthinkable," 178: "With respect to a person whose will has no fixed determinate character, it seems that the notion of autonomy or self-direction cannot find a grip."
4. Note that this argument could apply both at the level of a complete preference structure, or, more plausibly, at the level of a subset of a preference structure.
5. For the distinction between a person's substantial will and his Hobbesian (or "appetitive") will, see Cuypers, "Harry Frankfurt on the Will," 44–45.
6. For a discussion of a similar point see Bernard Berofsky, "Autonomy Without Free Will," in *Personal Autonomy*, ed. Taylor, 58–86.
7. For a discussion of this point see Frankfurt, "On the Necessity of Ideals," 111. Note that the sense of "identify" that is being used here is the colloquial sense of this term, rather than the philosophical sense as this is outlined in Chapters 3 and 4. Noting this is important, for some persons have conflated these terms to the detriment of their analysis of the latter. See, for example, Angela M. Smith, "Identification and Responsibility," in *Moral Responsibility and Ontology*, ed. Ton van den Beld, 239 (Dordrecht: Kluwer Academic Publishers, 2000).
8. The answer that a person must be sufficiently bound by the internal constraints of the contours of his self to be self-directed, autonomous, is parallel to H. Tristram Engelhardt's views concerning the way in which bioethical decisions can still be made in a context in which there is no clearly established objective morality. See his *The Foundations of Bioethics*, especially chap. 1, 2.
9. Frankfurt, "Autonomy, Necessity, and Love," 132. Note that recognizing that Frankfurt is here writing of autonomy and not of identification is compatible with the claims outlined in Chapter 3.
10. Ibid., 132.
11. Frankfurt, "On the Necessity of Ideals," 113.
12. Ibid., 113.
13. Frankfurt, "Rationality and the Unthinkable," 187.

186   *Notes*

14. Harry G. Frankfurt, "The Importance of What We Care About," 86. See also Bernard Williams, "Moral Incapacity," in *Making Sense of Humanity and Other Philosophical Papers 1982–1993*, ed. Bernard Williams, 46–55 (Cambridge: Cambridge University Press). For a comparison of the incapacities discussed by Frankfurt and Williams, see Gary Watson, "Volitional Necessities," in *Contours of Agency*, eds. Buss and Overton, 143–146.
15. Frankfurt, "On the Necessity of Ideals," 114.
16. It is thus clear that, as was argued in Chapter 3, the concepts of identification and autonomy are distinct for Frankfurt, since the conditions for a person identifying with her effective first-order desires are less stringent than for her to be autonomous with respect to them. This is because in addition to volitionally endorsing her effective first-order desires and being satisfied with this endorsement, as is required for a person to identify with them on Frankfurt's view, to be autonomous with respect to such desires a person's volitional endorsement of them must also stem from the essential nature of her substantial will. That is to say, to be autonomous with respect to an effective first-order desire on Frankfurt's view it must be motivating the person concerning to perform an action out of volitional necessity, or to refrain from performing one owing to its unthinkability.
17. Frankfurt, "Autonomy, Necessity, and Love," 132.
18. Ibid., 132.
19. Frankfurt, "Rationality and the Unthinkable," 183.
20. For a criticism of Frankfurt's account of autonomy as being not an account of autonomy but an account of authenticity, see Velleman, "Identification and Identity," 97–98. See also Chapter 2 for a discussion of autonomy and authenticity.
21. Frankfurt, "On the Necessity of Ideals," 114.
22. Ibid., 114.
23. Ibid., 114.
24. Theodore Sturgeon, "The Dark Room," in *The Golden Helix*, ed. Theodore Sturgeon, 191–227 (Garden City, NY: Nelson Doubleday, 1979).
25. Noggle, "Autonomy and the Paradox of Self-Creation," 87.
26. Marilyn Friedman, "Autonomy and the Split-Level Self," *Southern Journal of Philosophy* 24, no. 1 (1986): 24.
27. Stefaan E. Cuypers, "Autonomy Beyond Voluntarism: In Defense of Hierarchy," *Canadian Journal of Philosophy* 30, no. 2 (2000): 230.
28. Christman, "Introduction," 10. Note that Christman is mistaken to hold that autonomy is a property of desires, instead of a property of persons with respect to their desires.
29. Note that this is not to imply in itself that any of the three authors noted previously make either of these mistakes.
30. Although it is clear that Christman believes that autonomy is a property of person's psychological states or processes (for he writes of persons' desires being autonomous) it is not so clear that Friedman and Cuypers share this assumption—indeed, both appear to hold the correct view that autonomy is a property of persons with respect to their desires, actions, and so on. See here Friedman, "Autonomy and Male Dominance," 155; and Cuypers, *Self-Identity and Personal Autonomy*, chap. 4.
31. For further discussion of a related point see Noggle, "Autonomy and the Paradox of Self-Creation," 103.
32. For further discussion of this point—although one that is mistakenly cashed out in terms of identification—see Taylor, "Identification and Quasi-Desires," 111–136.

33. For an outline of the debate, see Cuypers, *Self-Identity and Personal Autonomy*, chap. 1.
34. Note that this account of what conditions must be met for a person to be autonomous with respect to her decisions will be supplemented by the Tracing Condition, to capture those cases when a person decides to make her decisions through a decision-making procedure that she is not yet satisfied with.
35. Berofsky, "Autonomy Without Free Will," 64.
36. Ibid., 64.
37. Marina A. L. Oshana, for example, holds that "Economic autonomy is a requirement of personal autonomy," following Diana Tietjens Meyers's claim that "People seek economic self-sufficiency to rule out the possibility that others might gain control over them through their needs. If one can take care of oneself, one is beholden to no one [sic]—neither to the state or to any other individual." (Oshana, *Personal Autonomy in Society*, 87; Meyers, *Self, Society, and Personal Choice*, 12.) Three points are worth noting here. First, in claiming that economic self-sufficiency is a requirement of personal autonomy Oshana is making a claim that is stronger than the usual claim that a person's poverty can compromise her autonomy, for, according to Oshana, being free from poverty is a necessary condition for being autonomous to begin with. Second, Oshana and Meyers here confuse being at risk of being subject to the control of other persons with being subject to the control of other persons—and while the latter would serve to compromise autonomy the former does not. Finally, if Oshana and Meyers are correct autonomy will be a very rare condition indeed, enjoyed only by persons who are independently wealthy or who live self-sufficient lives, including providing their own food and clothing.
38. See, for example, Hughes, "Exploitation, Autonomy, and the Case for Organ Sales," 89–95.
39. Raz, *The Morality of Freedom*, 374.
40. Ibid., 374.
41. See Taylor, "Autonomy, Inducements, and Organ Sales," 152–154.
42. A possible exception to this would be a person who is so impoverished that she lacks either the time or the energy, or both, to do anything other than attempt to remain alive. Such a person's poverty would then render her less autonomous than her wealthier counterparts, insofar as it would render her unable even to meet the minimal conditions for her to be exercising her autonomy. Yet, even so, even such a person would still possess the capacity for autonomy.
43. Mills, "Choice and Circumstance," 162.
44. Cherry, *Kidney for Sale by Owner*, 92.
45. For an extensive discussion of such constraints see Christman, "Liberalism, Autonomy, and Self-Transformation," 190–194.
46. This does not imply that a person's death is a harm to her. For arguments for this Epicurean conclusion, see Stephen Rosenbaum, "Epicurus and Annihilation," *The Philosophical Quarterly* 39, no. 154 (1989): 81–90.
47. Carolyn M. Stone, "Autonomy, Emotions, and Desires: Some Problems Concerning R. F. Dearden's Account of Autonomy," *Journal of Philosophy of Education* 24, no. 2 (1990): 276. Quoted in Aharon Aviram, "Autonomy and Commitment: Compatible Ideals," *Journal of Philosophy of Education* 29, no. 1 (1995): 61.
48. Allen Buchanan, "Assessing the Communitarian Critique of Liberalism," *Ethics* 99, no. 4 (1989): 868. Quoted in Andrew Mason, "Community and Autonomy: Logically Incompatible Values?" *Analysis* 51, no. 3 (1991): 162. As Mason notes, Buchanan does not endorse this argument.

49. This claim is considered at length in Mason, "Community and Autonomy," 160–166.

50. This could be for one of two reasons. First, the person in question might, for example, wish to be married to a particular person, and so when he autonomously marries the person in question this will itself enhance the instrumental value of his autonomy for him. Second, the person might believe that whereas he does not wish to be tempted to continue to date, he realizes that, were he not to be married, he would be tempted to do so. For such a person getting married will serve as a protective constraint against the possibility of autonomy undermining (as ambivalence inducing) temptation.

51. A similar response is offered by Mason in response to argument that autonomy and community are incompatible values (Mason, "Community and Autonomy," 162). In this way, then, such unfortunate commitments would affect the autonomy of those subject to them in the same way as poverty would typically affect the autonomy of those subject to it.

52. For further discussion of this see Taylor, "Autonomy, Duress, and Coercion," 152–155.

## NOTES TO CHAPTER 8

1. Samuel D. Warren and Louis D. Brandeis, "The Right to Privacy [the Implicit Made Explicit]," in *Philosophical Dimensions of Privacy: An Anthology*, ed. Ferdinand D. Schoeman, 75 (Cambridge: Cambridge University Press, 1984). The claim that a violation of one's privacy will also serve to undermine one's autonomy is repeated almost *ad nauseum* in the literature on privacy. See, for example, Joel Feinberg, "Autonomy," 53, n. 44; Joseph Kupfer, "Privacy, Autonomy, and Self-Concept," *American Philosophical Quarterly* 24, no. 1 (1987): 81–89; Richard Lippke, "Work, Privacy and Autonomy," *Public Affairs Quarterly* 3, no. 2 (1989): 49; Margaret Falls-Corbitt and F. Michael McClain, "God and Privacy," *Faith and Philosophy* 9, no. 3 (1992): 369–386; Mark Tunick, "Does Privacy Undermine Community?" *Journal of Value Inquiry* 35, no. 4 (2001): 529–531; Elizabeth L. Beardsley, "Privacy: Autonomy and Selective Disclosure," in *Nomos XIII: Privacy*, eds. J. Roland Pennock and John W. Chapman, 56–70 (New York: Atherton Press, 1971); Hyman Gross, "Privacy and Autonomy," in *Nomos XIII: Privacy*, eds. Pennock and Chapman, 169–181; Stanley I. Benn, "Privacy, Freedom, and Respect for Persons," in *Philosophical Dimensions of Privacy*, ed. Schoeman, 223–244; Charles Fried, "Privacy [A Moral Analysis]," in *Philosophical Dimensions of Privacy*, ed. Schoeman, 203–222; Ruth Gavison, "Privacy and the Limits of Law," in *Philosophical Dimensions of Privacy*, ed. Schoeman, 346–402; Robert S. Gerstein, "Intimacy and Privacy," in *Philosophical Dimensions of Privacy*, ed. Schoeman, 265–271.

2. Sabine Michalowski, *Medical Confidentiality and Crime* (Aldershot, England: Ashgate Publishing, 2003), 17.

3. James W. Jones, "Limits of Confidentiality: Disclosure of HIV Seropositivity," *Journal of Vascular Surgery* 38, no. 6 (2003): 1443. See also B. Woodward, "Confidentiality, Consent and Autonomy in the Physician–Patient Relationship," *Health Care Analysis* 9, no. 3 (2001): 337–351.

4. Recall here Arpaly's example (discussed in Chapter 2) of the thief who fails to respect his victim's autonomy by stealing from her but who does not thereby render her less able to exercise her autonomy. As was noted both in Chapter 2 and also in Chapter 6, while Arpaly is correct to hold that reducing the

number of options that a person has does not render her less autonomous *simpliciter*, this does not support the conclusion that she wishes to draw concerning normative moral autonomy.

5. For example, Joel Feinberg claims that "spying in the personal realm would be an outrageous violation of privacy, and hence of personal autonomy" ("Autonomy," 53, n. 44). Similarly, Richard Lippke argues that invasions of privacy will necessarily have "debilitating effects on . . . autonomy" ("Work, Privacy and Autonomy," 49).

6. Gross, "Privacy and Autonomy," 169, 173.

7. Fried, "Privacy [A Moral Analysis]," 209. See also Kupfer, "Privacy, Autonomy, and Self-Concept," 81–89.

8. Lisa Schwartz, Paul Preece, Ron Hendry, *Medical Ethics: A Case-Based Approach* (Oxford: Saunders Ltd, 2002), 45.

9. Chris Hackler, *Health Care for an Aging Population* (Albany, NY: SUNY Press, 1994), 156.

10. Falls-Corbitt and McClain have offered a version of this argument in "God and Privacy," 370–371.

11. Judith Jarvis Thomson, "The Right to Privacy," in *Philosophical Dimensions of Privacy*, ed. Schoeman, 288, n. 1. Although Thomson is here addressing the question of what it is to have a right to privacy her argument works equally well against attempts to analyze the concept of privacy in terms of control.

12. This inherently normative account of privacy is similar to that offered by William A. Parent, "Recent Work on the Concept of Privacy," *American Philosophical Quarterly* 20, no. 4 (1983): 341–355. Alan Westin gives anthropological evidence for the essential normativity of privacy in "The Origins of Modern Claims to Privacy," in *Philosophical Dimensions of Privacy*, ed. Schoeman, 58–66. It should be noted that this is an account of what it is for something to *be* private. For an account of what it is for someone to enjoy privacy (or to enjoy the right to privacy), an additional criterion must be added, namely, that one's privacy *actually does* remain inviolate.

13. Applying it to Thomson's example shows that this normative account of privacy is not linked to control. Unlike the case in which privacy is defined in terms of control, on this account of privacy Thomson's neighbor's privacy is not violated when the X-ray device is trained on her house because even when this is done Thomson does not actually gain access to any information that her neighbor would be justified in refusing her access to. It is only when Thomson actually uses the device (and so actually gains access to information that she may be excluded from) that she violates her neighbor's privacy.

14. It should be noted that these arguments do not depend upon one's accepting the characterization of privacy given previously. Indeed, none of the positive arguments that follow need rely on any particular characterization of privacy in order to be persuasive.

15. Kupfer, "Privacy, Autonomy, and Self-Concept," 82.

16. Ibid. Although in his working definition of privacy Kupfer characterizes it in terms of control, his arguments linking privacy and autonomy do not depend on this, for they could be made equally well using the normative account of privacy outlined previously. Thus, for example, insofar as it is instrumentally valuable in being required for the development of autonomy that a child enjoy privacy with respect to information concerning her psychological state, insofar as autonomy is valued it would be unjustified for one to seek to violate the child's privacy with respect to her psychological state. Similarly, if a person is justified in withholding from others her moral and political views, then she should enjoy privacy with respect to her deliberations concerning

these when she wishes to engage in self-reflection. Since Kupfer's arguments do not rest on defining privacy in terms of control, they are not susceptible to Thomson-style counterexamples.

17. Ibid.
18. Jean Piaget, *The Moral Judgment of the Child* (New York: Basic Books, 1966); Victor Tausk, "On the Origin of the 'Influencing Machine' in Schizophrenia," *Psychoanalytic Quarterly* 2 (1933): 519–556. Cited by Kupfer, "Privacy, Autonomy, and Self-Concept," 88.
19. Kupfer, "Privacy, Autonomy, and Self-Concept," 82.
20. Ibid., 84.
21. Benn, "Privacy, Freedom, and Respect for Persons," 241.
22. Versions of this argument have been proposed by Benn, "Privacy, Freedom, and Respect for Persons," 241, and Edward J. Bloustein, "Privacy as an Aspect of Human Dignity: An Answer to Dean Prosser," in *Philosophical Dimensions of Privacy*, ed. Schoeman, 188. A similar argument has also been offered by James Rachels, who argued that the different relationships that persons have with others are defined by the different patterns of behavior that persons exhibit with each other. Rachels argues the possession of control over the knowledge that persons have of one constitutes (at least in part) what it is for one to be able to autonomously control the type of relationships that she has with others. Rachels argues that since this is so, if one lacks such control over information about oneself—if one lacks the ability to keep some information private, or to choose to make it public—then one will also lack a degree of autonomy with respect to the types of relationships that one has with others. James Rachels, "Why Privacy Is Important," *Philosophy and Public Affairs* 4, no. 4 (1975): 323–33. See also Schwartz, Preece, and Hendry, *Medical Ethics*, 45.
23. Daniel C. Dennett, *Elbow Room: The Varieties of Free Will Worth Wanting* (Cambridge: MIT Press, 1984), 52.
24. This model of motivation has been outlined by Robert Audi in his "The Structure of Motivation," *Pacific Philosophical Quarterly* 61, no. 3 (1980): 258–275 and by Robert Noggle in his "Kantian Respect and Particular Persons," *Canadian Journal of Philosophy* 26, no. 3 (1999): 459–460.
25. Bernard Williams, "A Critique of Utilitarianism," in *Utilitarianism: For and Against*, eds. J. J. C. Smart and Bernard Williams, 113 (Cambridge: Cambridge University Press, 1973). For a discussion of this distinction between the pro-attitudes that are shared by all persons and those that are relative to the motivational-sets of particular individuals in the context of the distinction between a person's agential motivations and those that she is autonomous with respect to, see Chapter 3.
26. As it stands this account of human motivation has been simplified, for it will not be the case that a person's first-order desires will stem directly from the combination of one of her core motivations with a belief. Instead, most of her first-order desires will stem from the combination of a preexisting desire that specifies its object in more or less precise terms and that had a core motivation-belief pair in its ancestry. For the sake of simplicity, however, this complication will be ignored in the following discussion, for it does not affect the substance of this account of how a violation of one's privacy might undermine one's autonomy. For further discussion of this point—albeit in the context of a discussion of identification—see Taylor, "Identification and Quasi-Desires," 111–136.
27. Or believes that he is likely to be under observation.
28. Alternatively, this couple might have believed that they were being watched. In this case they would not have suffered from their autonomy being compromised for the reason given in the second condition.

29. She will, however, still enjoy a degree of autonomy with respect to her actions because what actions she performs and how she performs them will not be entirely under the control of those who place her under this form of duress. For a discussion of this point, see James W. Child, "Specific Commands, General Rules, and Degrees of Autonomy," *Canadian Journal of Law and Jurisprudence* 8, no. 2 (1995): 245–58. It should also be noted that she will also be autonomous with respect to her decisions and her effective first-order desires. Unlike situations where a person's privacy is covertly violated, a person whose privacy is overtly violated will make her decisions knowing that she is being watched. If she thus decides to conform her actions to what she believes to be the values of her observers, then she will be autonomous with respect to this decision. However, since the intentional objects of the desires that she accordingly decides to satisfy will be "to perform those actions that will avoid the disapprobation of my observers," she will have ceded control over what actions she performs to her observers. And, since this is so, even though she might be fully autonomous with respect to her decisions and her effective first-order desires to perform these actions she will not be fully autonomous with respect to the actions themselves. For a discussion of this point see Taylor, "Autonomy, Duress, and Coercion," 152–155.
30. For a discussion of this, see Linda Beecham, "BMA Annual Representative Meeting: Debate Needed on Balance Between Patient Confidentiality and Needs of Research," *British Medical Journal* 329, no. 7457 (2004), 72.

## NOTES TO CHAPTER 9

1. Beauchamp and Childress, *The Principles of Biomedical Ethics*, 77.
2. R. R. Faden and T. L. Beauchamp, *A History and Theory of Informed Consent* (New York: Oxford University Press, 1986), 235; S. Appelbaum, C. W. Lidz, and A. Meisel, *Informed Consent* (New York: Oxford University Press, 1987), 3.
3. See *Canterbury v. Spence*, 464 F2d 784 (DC Circ, 1972).
4. For further discussion of this point, see Chapter 1.
5. For an extensive discussion of this point see Alan Merry and Alexander McCall Smith, *Errors, Medicine and the Law* (Cambridge: Cambridge University Press, 2001), 152–175.
6. Thomas May, *Bioethics in a Liberal Society* (Baltimore: The Johns Hopkins University Press, 2002), 39.
7. Faden and Beauchamp, *A History and Theory of Informed Consent*, 37–38. For a further discussion of the relationship between autonomy, manipulation, and deception, see Chapter 1.
8. Note that this claim is compatible with accepting the autonomy-based justification for the doctrine of informed consent that will be developed next.
9. *Cobbs v. Grant*, 502 P.2d 1, 12 (1972).
10. At this juncture, then, it seems that if a healthcare provider such as Grant fails to inform his patients of the risks associated with their medical treatment, he will wrong them because this puts their well-being at risk.
11. Beauchamp and Childress, *Principles of Biomedical Ethics*, 58.
12. Note that in assessing whether or not a certain action was a prudent one for a person to perform would be assessed on the basis of whether it is *likely* to be one that will enable her to achieve the ends that she intends to achieve through its performance. This part of the response to the above objection to the argument against the view that concern for autonomy is not the ethical foundation of informed consent represents a modification of an earlier

response to it, in which it was argued that this objection implausibly construes autonomy as a success condition. See James Stacey Taylor, "Autonomy and Informed Consent: A Much Misunderstood Relationship," *Journal of Value Inquiry* 38, no. 3 (2004): 388. This modification is made in response to a criticism of this earlier response that was leveled against it by Jukka Varelius, "On Taylor on Autonomy and Informed Consent," *Journal of Value Inquiry* 40, no 4 (2006): 455.

13. Note that the point of this example is independent of accepting the religious presuppositions that lie behind it. It, rather than the other obvious example that could make the same point (Oedipus's lack of blameworthiness for unwittingly marrying his mother), was chosen because Jesus, unlike Oedipus, himself makes the point that his executioners are not to be blamed for what they do owing to their ignorance of the most morally salient intensional description of their actions. ("Father, forgive them for they know not what they do." Luke 23:34) For discussions of the ways in which a person's culpability for her actions need not track her autonomy with respect to them see Marina A. L. Oshana, "The Misguided Marriage of Responsibility and Autonomy," *The Journal of Ethics* 6, no. 3 (2002): 261–280; McKenna, "The Relationship Between Autonomous and Morally Responsible Agency," 205–234.

14. Note that as is now generally recognized in the philosophical literature on well-being a person's satisfaction of her desires need not contribute to her achieving her goals but could even impair this.

15. This is the first of the two ways in which a person might fail to respect the autonomy of another that were outlined in the previous chapter.

16. For further discussion of points related to this, see Taylor, "Autonomy, Duress, and Coercion," 127–155, and the discussion of self-imposed constraints in Chapter 7.

17. Varelius, "On Taylor on Autonomy and Informed Consent," 454. The fourth view that Varelius identifies and his objection to it will be discussed in n.27.

18. Ibid., 454.

19. Ibid.

20. Ibid. Varelius's purported counterexample is underdescribed, for it is not clear whether the irresistible desire in question is a strongly irresistible desire (i.e., one whose motivational efficacy would move its possessor to satisfy it immediately, whenever it took hold), or a weakly irresistible desire (i.e., one whose motivational efficacy could be resisted by its possessor for a while, and so she could choose when to satisfy it). (For a further discussion of this distinction see Taylor, "Willing Addicts, Unwilling Addicts, and Acting of One's Own Free Will," 242–244. Note, though, that the discussion in this paper mistakenly conflates a person's identifying with her effective first-order desires with her being autonomous with respect to them.) If the desire in question is a weakly irresistible desire, then insofar as it will be the agent who decides when and where to satisfy it, she would still be autonomous with respect to her decision to do so and her consequent actions, on the account of autonomy outlined in Chapter 1. (Although since being subject to this desire would render her situation a Frankfurtian situation of Type A her possession of it would reduce the instrumental value of her autonomy to her.) Since this is so, Varelius's counterexample requires that the irresistible desire in question be a strongly irresistible desire.

21. The example of a man who has been reduced to the status of a contented infant as a result of an accident is borrowed from Thomas Nagel, who uses it for a different purpose. See his "Death," in *The Metaphysics of Death*, ed. John Martin Fischer, 65 (Stanford, CA: Stanford University Press, 1993).

22. Varelius, "On Taylor on Autonomy and Informed Consent," 458.

23. Taylor, "Autonomy and Informed Consent," 386.
24. Varelius, "Taylor on Autonomy and Informed Consent," 455.
25. Note that the argument offered previously has been modified from its original version to accommodate Varelius's concerns regarding autonomy as a success concept.
26. Varelius, "On Taylor on Autonomy and Informed Consent,"456. Although Varelius is here mistakenly treating autonomy as a property of decisions instead of as a property of persons with respect to their decisions this error does not affect his argument.
27. Varelius's objection to (iv) can be met in the same way that his objection to (iii) can be met. Varelius objects to view (iv) that "maintaining that respect for patient's [sic] autonomy means providing her with relevant information would be self-defeating as a defense of the conventional view about the relationship between autonomy and informed consent." The reason that this view was held to be self-defeating as a defense of the view that concern for informed consent was based on concern for patient autonomy was that an account of what information would be "relevant" in this context would be indexed to the desires and values of the patient concerned. Thus, rather than exhibiting concern for her autonomy the provision of such information would instead evince concern for her well-being. (Taylor, "Autonomy and Informed Consent," 391.) Varelius objects to this on the grounds that no distinction can be made between "acting in response to the value of autonomy per se and acting in order to help the patient in the pursuit of her desires and values," for he believes that he has shown (in his objection to view [ii]) that "mere non-interference with [the] decisions and actions of others, does not amount to respecting their autonomy." (Varelius, "On Taylor on Autonomy and Informed Consent," 457.) However, since Varelius's objection to (ii) is mistaken, so too is his objection to (iv).
28. Varelius offers a version of this argument when he objects to view (iv), outlined previously.
29. Note that this thus does not require that a healthcare professional work to maximize the instrumental value of their patients' autonomy to them through medical means, even if they request it. A healthcare professional's duty to respect the instrumental value of his patients' autonomy through securing or enhancing it for them through his craft does not require, for example, that he prescribe them performance-enhancing drugs, even if such drugs would indeed enhance the instrumental value of the autonomy of the patients who requested it to them.
30. In fairness to Varelius, it should be noted that this is a conclusion that he, too, would endorse—even though his own arguments do not serve to justify it.

## NOTES TO CHAPTER 10

1. Or, more accurately, that autonomy has instrumental value to *most* persons. Some persons might desire to live entirely subject to the direction of others, and, if these people are correct to believe that this would be the most appropriate life for them to live, their autonomy would not even be of instrumental value to them.
2. The temptation to infer from the fact that the exercise of autonomy is instrumental in enabling persons to attempt to satisfy their desires or fulfill their goals to the conditional claim that if the value that autonomy is instrumental in securing is that of human well-being then the appropriate analysis of well-being will be a preference-satisfaction or interest-fulfillment account should be resisted, for two reasons. First, that autonomy is of instrumental value in this way is compatible with other analyses of well-being, such as, for

example, hedonism. Second, it will be argued next that there is good reason to reject preference- or interest-based analyses of well-being.

3. That autonomy has instrumental, rather than intrinsic, value has been argued for by Christopher Tollefsen, "*Sic Et Non*: Some Disputed Questions in Reproductive Ethics," in *Handbook of Bioethics: Taking Stock of the Field from a Philosophical Perspective*, ed. George Khushf, 404 (Dordrecht: Springer, 2004).

4. As James Griffin puts it, "Even if you convince me that, as my personal despot, you would produce more desirable consciousness for me than I do for myself, I shall want to go on being my own master, at least as long as your record would not be much better than mine. . . . And I should prefer it. . . because it would make for a better life for me to live." James Griffin, *Well-Being: Its Meaning, Measurement, and Moral Importance* (Oxford: Clarendon Press, 1986), 9.

5. Friedman, "Autonomy and Male Dominance," 167; that the view that autonomy is of intrinsic value is in accord with "the prevailing strength of philosophical opinion" is noted by Robert Young, "The Value of Autonomy," *The Philosophical Quarterly* 32, no. 126 (1982): 35. A similar point is made concerning the intrinsic value that is accorded autonomy by medical ethicists by James Wilson, "Is Respect for Autonomy Defensible?" *Journal of Medical Ethics* 33, no. 6 (2007): 353–356. The bioethical view that autonomy has intrinsic value is prominently endorsed by Ronald Dworkin, *Life's Dominion: An Argument about Abortion, Euthanasia, and Individual Freedom* (New York: Vintage, 1994).

6. Hurka, "Why Value Autonomy?" 366.

7. Ibid., 366.

8. Ibid., 366.

9. Ibid., 368–369.

10. Ibid., 368.

11. Ibid., 370.

12. Mills, "Choice and Circumstance," 158.

13. Hurka, "Why Value Autonomy?" 373.

14. Ibid., 372, 374–375.

15. Mills, "Choice and Circumstance," 159.

16. This example is Hurka's own: "Why Value Autonomy?" 366.

17. The background assumption behind these examples is that absent the manipulations of Iago, Othello would be fully autonomous with respect to his desires and his actions.

18. This example is a version of the "experience machine" example developed by Robert Nozick, *Anarchy, State, and Utopia* (Oxford: Blackwell, 1974), 42–45.

19. Joel Feinberg, "Harm to Others," in Fischer, ed., *The Metaphysics of Death*, 179.

20. W. D. Ross, *Foundations of Ethics* (Oxford: Clarendon Press, 1939), 300; Feinberg, "Harm to Others," 177.

21. Ibid., 178. An extensive criticism of Feinberg's desire-fulfillment account of well-being has been offered by Douglas Portmore, in the context of arguing that Feinberg's anti-hedonistic arguments fail to establish that posthumous harm is possible. Douglas Portmore, "Desire Fulfillment and Posthumous Harm," *American Philosophical Quarterly* 44, no. 1 (2007): 27–38. For further objections to Feinberg's use of this anti-hedonistic argument to establish the possibility of posthumous harm, see James Stacey Taylor, "The Myth of Posthumous Harm," *American Philosophical Quarterly* 42, no. 4 (2005): 311–322.

22. Feinberg, "Harm to Others," 181–182.
23. Ibid., 182.
24. George Berkeley, *A Treatise Concerning the Principles of Human Knowledge* (La Vergne, TN: Filiquarian, Inc., 2007), sect. 1.
25. It is true that a person subject to deception will suffer from a diminution in autonomy with respect to her decisions and actions that she consequently performs. But to hold that this in itself will make the life of a person so deceived worse than it otherwise would be, would be to beg the question against the view that autonomy is not of intrinsic value.
26. For a discussion of this point in relation to Cartesian skepticism, see O. K. Bouwsma, "Descartes' Evil Genius," *The Philosophical Review* 58, no. 2 (1949): 141–151.
27. Note that to claim that this woman was harmed by the collapse of her projects even though this never came to affect her experiences is not the same as claiming that she was harmed by the collapse of her projects even though she never came to know either of the collapse of the consequent harm, for one could deny the old saw that "what you don't know doesn't hurt you" without denying that an event must have affected a person's experiences to affect her well-being. Since the proponent of a defensible account of hedonism would indeed deny the former claim while affirming the latter, and Feinberg's Case A is intended to be a counterexample to hedonism, view (iii) is construed in the way that fits best with the hedonism that is Feinberg's target.
28  For a discussion of this point see Geoffrey Scarre, "Archaeology and Respect for the Dead," *Journal of Applied Philosophy* 20, no. 3 (2003): 237–249.
29. That Feinberg would certainly claim this for his Case A was developed as part of an argument to show that posthumous harm is possible.
30. Feinberg, "Harm to Others," 182.
31. George Pitcher, "The Misfortunes of the Dead," in *The Metaphysics of Death*, ed. John Martin Fischer, 168.
32. Ibid., 168.
33. This counterfactual view of harm has been outlined and defended by Thomas Nagel, "Death," 65–66.
34. A more complete argument for this conclusion is developed in Taylor, "The Myth of Posthumous Harm," 311–322.
35. Barbara Baum Levenbook, "Harming Someone After His Death," *Ethics* 94, no. 3 (1984), 416–417.
36. Joan Callahan, "On Harming the Dead," *Ethics* 97, no. 2 (1987): 342–343.
37. Ibid., 343.
38. Dworkin, *The Theory and Practice of Autonomy*, 80.
39. See, for example, Jonathan Glover, *Causing Death and Saving Lives* (New York: Penguin, 1977), chap. 5.
40. See, for example, Susan J. Brison, "The Autonomy Defense of Free Speech," *Ethics* 108, no. 2 (1998): 312–339.
41. See, for example, George Sher, *Beyond Neutrality: Perfectionism and Politics* (Cambridge: Cambridge University Press, 1997), esp. chap. 4.
42. See P. Allmark, "Choosing Health and the Inner Citadel," *Journal of Medical Ethics* 32, no. 1 (2006): 3–6.
43. *Bigelow v. Virginia*, 421 U.S. 809 (1975).
44. *Virginia State Bd. of Pharmacy v. Virginia Citizens Consumer Council*, 425 U.S. 748 (1976).
45. It was on this basis that certain Native American groups objected to the Patient Self-Determination Act that became effective in the United States in 1991. See James Stacey Taylor, "Autonomy and Informed Consent on the Navajo Reservation," *Journal of Social Philosophy* 35, no. 4 (2004): 506.

46. See Smith, "The Pre-eminence of Autonomy in Bioethics," 182–195.
47. Hurka, "Why Value Autonomy?" 363.
48. Although given Hurka's view of autonomy it is clear that he considers the removal of such options a violation of autonomy in that it will, on his view, render her agency less effective.
49. This argument is discussed more fully in Taylor, *Stakes and Kidneys*, chap. 5.
50. Such as, for example, the possibility that value is an agent-relative rather than an agent-neutral concept, and the corresponding issues of value incommensurability.

## NOTES TO THE CONCLUSION

1. For a discussion of the Navajo's metaphysical beliefs and their implications for the implementation of the Patient Self-Determination Act among them see Taylor, "Autonomy and Informed Consent on the Navajo Reservation," 506–516.

# Bibliography

Ainslie, Donald C. "Bioethics and the Problem of Pluralism." In *Bioethics*, edited by Ellen Frankel Paul, Fred Dycus Miller Jr., Jeffrey Paul, 1–28. Cambridge: Cambridge University Press, 2002.

Allmark, P. "Choosing Health and the Inner Citadel." *Journal of Medical Ethics* 32, no. 1 (2006): 3–6.

Anderson, Scott A. "Prostitution and Sexual Autonomy: Making Sense of the Prohibition of Prostitution." *Ethics* 112, no. 4 (2002): 748–780.

Appelbaum, S., C. W. Lidz, and A. Meisel. *Informed Consent.* New York: Oxford University Press, 1987.

Arpaly, Nomy. "Responsibility, Applied Ethics, and Complex Autonomy Theories." In *Personal Autonomy: New Essays on Personal Autonomy and Its Role in Contemporary Moral Philosophy*, edited by James Stacey Taylor, 162–180. Cambridge: Cambridge University Press, 2005.

————. *Unprincipled Virtue: An Inquiry Into Moral Agency.* New York: Oxford University Press, 2003.

Athanassoulis, Nafsika. "Unusual Requests and the Doctor-Patient Relationship." *Journal of Value Inquiry* 40, nos. 2–3 (2006): 259–278.

Audi, Robert. "The Structure of Motivation." *Pacific Philosophical Quarterly* 61, no. 3 (1980): 258–275.

Aviram, Aharon. "Autonomy and Commitment: Compatible Ideals." *Journal of Philosophy of Education* 29, no. 1 (1995): 61–79.

Bauer, M. *The Field Guide to Psychiatric Assessment and Treatment.* Philadelphia: Lippincott/Williams and Wilkins, 2003.

Beardsley, Elizabeth L. "Privacy: Autonomy and Selective Disclosure." In *Nomos XIII: Privacy*, edited by J. Roland Pennock and John W. Chapman, 56–70. New York: Atherton Press, 1971.

Beauchamp, Tom L. "Who Deserves Autonomy, and Whose Autonomy Deserves Respect?" In *Personal Autonomy: New Essays on Personal Autonomy and Its Role in Contemporary Moral Philosophy*, edited by James Stacey Taylor, 310–329. Cambridge: Cambridge University Press, 2005.

Beauchamp, Tom L., and James F. Childress. *Principles of Biomedical Ethics.* Fifth edition. Oxford: Oxford University Press, 2001.

Beecham, Linda. "BMA Annual Representative Meeting: Debate Needed on Balance Between Patient Confidentiality and Needs of Research." *British Medical Journal* 329 (2004): 72.

Benn, Stanley, I. "Privacy, Freedom, and Respect for Persons." In *Philosophical Dimensions of Privacy: An Anthology*, edited by Ferdinand D. Schoeman, 223–244. Cambridge: Cambridge University Press, 1984.

Benson, Paul. "Feminist Intuitions and the Normative Substance of Autonomy." In *Personal Autonomy: New Essays on Personal Autonomy and Its Role in*

*Contemporary Moral Philosophy*, edited by James Stacey Taylor, 124–142. Cambridge: Cambridge University Press, 2005.

———. "Taking Ownership: Authority and Voice in Autonomous Agency." In *Autonomy and the Challenges to Liberalism: New Essays*, edited by John Christman and Joel Anderson, 101–126. Cambridge: Cambridge University Press, 2005.

Berkeley, George. *A Treatise Concerning the Principles of Human Knowledge*. La Vergne, TN: Filiquarian, Inc., 2007.

Berlin, Isaiah. *Four Essays on Liberty*. Oxford: Oxford University Press, 1977.

Berofsky, Bernard. "Autonomy Without Free Will." In *Personal Autonomy: New Essays on Personal Autonomy and Its Role in Contemporary Moral Philosophy*, edited by James Stacey Taylor, 58–86. Cambridge: Cambridge University Press, 2005.

———. *Liberation from Self: A Theory of Personal Autonomy*. Cambridge: Cambridge University Press, 1995.

Bixby, Jerome. "It's a *Good* Life." In *Star of Stars*, edited by Frederik Pohl, 219–240. Garden City, NY: Doubleday, 1960.

Bloustein, Edward J. "Privacy as an Aspect of Human Dignity: An Answer to Dean Prosser." In *Philosophical Dimensions of Privacy: An Anthology*, edited by Ferdinand D. Schoeman, 156–202. Cambridge: Cambridge University Press, 1984.

Blumberg, Henry, David Rimland, Donna Carroll, Pamela Terry, and Kaye Wachsmuth. "Rapid Development of Ciprofloxacin Resistance in Methicillin-Susceptable and –Resistant Staphylococcus aureus." *Journal of Infectious Diseases* 163, no. 6 (1991): 1279–1285.

Bouwsma, O. K. "Descartes' Evil Genius." *The Philosophical Review*, vol. 58, no. 2 (1949): 141–151.

Bratman, Michael. "Identification, Decision, and Treating as a Reason." *Philosophical Topics* 24, no. 2 (1996): 1–18.

———. "Planning Agency, Autonomous Agency." In *Personal Autonomy: New Essays on Personal Autonomy and Its Role in Contemporary Moral Philosophy*, edited by James Stacey Taylor, 33–57. Cambridge: Cambridge University Press, 2005.

———. "Reflection, Planning, and Temporally Extended Agency." In *Structures of Agency: Essays*, edited by Michael Bratman, 21–46. New York: Oxford University Press, 2007.

———. "Two Problems About Human Agency." In *Structures of Agency: Essays*, edited by Michael Bratman, 89–105. New York: Oxford University Press, 2007.

Brison, Susan J. "The Autonomy Defense of Free Speech." *Ethics* 108, no. 2 (1998): 312–339.

Buchanan, Allen. "Assessing the Communitarian Critique of Liberalism." *Ethics* 99, no. 4 (1989): 852–882.

Buss, Sarah. "Valuing Autonomy and Respecting Persons: Manipulation, Seduction, and the Basis of Moral Constraints." *Ethics* 113, no. 2 (2005): 195–235.

Callahan, Joan. "On Harming the Dead." *Ethics* 97, no. 2 (1987): 341–352.

Cherry, Mark J. *Kidney for Sale By Owner*. Georgetown: Georgetown University Press, 2005.

———. "Medical Innovation, Collapsing Goods, and the Moral Centrality of the Free Market." *Journal of Value Inquiry* 40, nos. 2–3 (2006): 209–226.

Child, James W. "Specific Commands, General Rules, and Degrees of Autonomy." *Canadian Journal of Law and Jurisprudence* 8, no. 2 (1995): 245–58.

Childress, James F. "The Place of Autonomy in Bioethics." *Hastings Center Report* 20, no. 1 (1990): 12–17.

Christman, John. "Autonomy and Personal History." *Canadian Journal of Philosophy* 21, no. 1 (1991): 1–24.

———. "Autonomy, Self-Knowledge, and Liberal Legitimacy." In *Autonomy and the Challenges to Liberalism: New Essays*, edited by John Christman and Joel Anderson, 330–357. Cambridge: Cambridge University Press, 2005.

———. "Defending Historical Autonomy: A Reply to Professor Mele." *Canadian Journal of Philosophy* 23, no. 2 (1993): 281–290.

———. "Introduction." In *The Inner Citadel: Essays on Individual Autonomy*, edited by John Christman, 3–23. New York: Oxford University Press, 1989.

———. "Liberalism and Individual Positive Freedom." *Ethics* 101, no. 2 (1991): 343–359.

———. "Liberalism, Autonomy, and Self-Transformation." *Social Theory and Practice* 27, no. 2 (2001): 185–206.

Christman, John, and Joel Anderson. "Introduction." In *Autonomy and the Challenges to Liberalism: New Essays*, edited by John Christman and Joel Anderson, 1–23. Cambridge: Cambridge University Press, 2005.

Coeckelbergh, Mark. *The Metaphysics of Autonomy: The Reconciliation of Ancient and Modern Ideals of the Person*. Basingstoke: Palgrave Macmillan, 2004.

Cuypers, Stefaan E. "Autonomy Beyond Voluntarism: In Defense of Hierarchy." *Canadian Journal of Philosophy* 30, no. 2 (2000): 225–256.

———. "Harry Frankfurt on the Will, Autonomy, and Necessity." *Ethical Perspectives* 5, no. 1 (1998): 44–52.

———. *Self-Identity and Personal Autonomy*. Aldershot, England: Ashgate Publishing, 2002.

Darwall, Stephen. "The Value of Autonomy and Autonomy of the Will." *Ethics* 116, no. 2 (2006): 264–284.

Davenport, John. *Will as Commitment and Resolve: An Existential Account of Creativity, Love, Virtue, and Happiness*. New York: Fordham University Press, 2007.

Dearden, R. F. "Autonomy and Education." In *Education and the Development of Reason*, edited by R. F. Dearden, P. H. Hirst, and R. S. Peters, 448–465. London: Routledge and Kegan Paul, 1972.

Dennett, Daniel C. *Elbow Room: The Varieties of Free Will Worth Wanting*. Cambridge: MIT Press, 1984.

Double, Richard. "Two Types of Autonomy Accounts." *Canadian Journal of Philosophy* 22, no. 1 (1992): 65–80.

Downie, R. S., and Elizabeth Tefler. "Autonomy." *Philosophy* 15 (1971): 293–301.

Dworkin, Gerald. "Autonomy and Behavior Control." *Hastings Center Report* 6, no. 1 (1976): 23–28.

———. "Markets and Morals: The Case for Organ Sales." In *Morality, Harm, and the Law*, edited by Gerald Dworkin, 155–161. Boulder, CO: Westview Press, 1994.

———. *The Theory and Practice of Autonomy*. Cambridge: Cambridge University Press, 1988.

Dworkin, Ronald. *Life's Dominion: An Argument About Abortion, Euthanasia, and Individual Freedom*. New York: Vintage, 1994.

Dwyer, Susan J. "The Many Faces of Autonomy." *The Philosophers' Magazine* 13 (2001): 40–41.

Ekstrom, Laura Waddell. "A Coherence Theory of Autonomy." *Philosophy and Phenomenological Research* 53, no. 3 (1993): 599–616.

Elster, Jon. *Sour Grapes: Studies in the Subversion of Rationality*. Cambridge: Cambridge University Press, 1983.

———. "Sour Grapes—Utilitarianism and the Genesis of Wants." In *The Inner Citadel: Essays on Individual Autonomy,* edited by John Christman, 170–188. New York: Oxford University Press, 1989.

Engelhardt, H. Tristram. *Foundations of Christian Bioethics.* Lisse, The Netherlands: Swets & Zeitlinger, 2000.

———. *The Foundations of Bioethics.* Second edition. New York: Oxford University Press, 1995.

———. "The Many Faces of Autonomy." *Health Care Analysis* 9, no. 3 (2001): 283–297.

Faden, R. R., and T. L. Beauchamp. *A History and Theory of Informed Consent.* New York: Oxford University Press, 1986.

Falls-Corbitt, Margaret, and F. Michael McClain. "God and Privacy." *Faith and Philosophy* 9, no. 3 (1992): 369–386.

Farsides, Bobbie, "Consent and the Capable Adult Patient—An Ethical Perspective: Consent and Patient Autonomy." In *Nursing Law and Ethics,* edited by John Tingle and Alan Cribb, 121–130. Second edition, Oxford: Blackwell: 2002.

Feinberg, Joel. "Autonomy." In *The Inner Citadel: Essays on Individual Autonomy,* edited by John Christman, 27–53. New York: Oxford University Press, 1989.

———. "The Idea of a Free Man." In *Educational Judgments: Papers in the Philosophy of Education,* edited by James F. Doyle, 142–169. London: Routledge, 1973.

———. "Harm to Others." In *The Metaphysics of Death,* edited by John Martin Fischer, 169–190. Stanford, CA: Stanford University Press, 1993.

Fowles, John. *The Collector.* Boston: Little, Brown and Company, 1963.

Frankfurt, Harry G. "Alternate Possibilities and Moral Responsibility." In *The Importance of What We Care About: Philosophical Essays,* edited by Harry G. Frankfurt, 1–10. Cambridge: Cambridge University Press, 1988.

———. "Autonomy, Necessity, and Love." In *Necessity, Volition, and Love,* edited by Harry G. Frankfurt, 129–141. Cambridge: Cambridge University Press, 1999.

———. "Coercion and Moral Responsibility." In *The Importance of What We Care About,* edited by Harry G. Frankfurt, 26–46. Cambridge: Cambridge University Press, 1988.

———. "Freedom of the Will and the Concept of a Person." In *The Importance of What We Care About: Philosophical Essays,* edited by Harry G. Frankfurt, 11–25. Cambridge: Cambridge University Press, 1988.

———. "Identification and Externality." In *The Importance of What We Care About,* edited by Harry G. Frankfurt, 58–68. Cambridge: Cambridge University Press, 1988.

———. "Identification and Wholeheartedness." In *The Importance of What We Care About,* edited by Harry G. Frankfurt, 159–176. Cambridge: Cambridge University Press, 1988.

———. "On the Necessity of Ideals." In *Necessity, Volition, and Love,* edited by Harry G. Frankfurt, 108–116. Cambridge: Cambridge University Press, 1999.

———. "Rationality and the Unthinkable." In *The Importance of What We Care About,* edited by Harry G. Frankfurt, 177–190. Cambridge: Cambridge University Press, 1988.

———. "Reply to Michael E. Bratman." In *Contours of Agency: Essays on Themes from Harry Frankfurt,* edited by Sarah Buss and Lee Overton, 86–95. Cambridge: MIT Press, 2002.

———. "The Faintest Passion." In *Necessity, Volition, and Love,* edited by Harry G. Frankfurt, 95–107. Cambridge: Cambridge University Press, 1999.

———. "The Importance of What We Care About." In *The Importance of What We Care About,* edited by Harry G. Frankfurt, 80–94. Cambridge: Cambridge University Press, 1988.

———. "Three Concepts of Free Action." In *The Importance of What We Care About*, edited by Harry G. Frankfurt, 47–57. Cambridge: Cambridge University Press, 1988.

Fried, Charles. "Privacy [A Moral Analysis]." In *Philosophical Dimensions of Privacy: An Anthology*, edited by Ferdinand D. Schoeman, 203–222. Cambridge: Cambridge University Press, 1984.

Friedman, Marilyn. "Autonomy and Male Dominance." In *Autonomy and the Challenges to Liberalism: New Essays*, edited by John Christman and Joel Anderson, 150–173. Cambridge: Cambridge University Press, 2005.

———. "Autonomy and the Split-Level Self." *Southern Journal of Philosophy* 24, no. 1 (1986): 19–35.

———. *Autonomy, Gender, Politics*. New York: Oxford University Press, 2003.

Frost, Rainer, "Political Liberty: Integrating Five Conceptions of Autonomy." In *Autonomy and the Challenges to Liberalism: New Essays*, edited by John Christman and Joel Anderson, 226–242. Cambridge: Cambridge University Press, 2005.

Gavison, Ruth. "Privacy and the Limits of Law." In *Philosophical Dimensions of Privacy: An* Anthology, edited by Ferdinand D. Schoeman, 346–402. Cambridge: Cambridge University Press, 1984.

Gerstein, Robert S. "Intimacy and Privacy." In *Philosophical Dimensions of Privacy: An Anthology*, edited by Ferdinand D. Schoeman, 265–271. Cambridge: Cambridge University Press, 1984.

Gilligan, Carol. *In a Different Voice*. Cambridge: Harvard University Press, 1982.

Gillon, R. "Ethics Needs Principles—Four Can Encompass the Rest—and Respect for Autonomy Should Be 'First Among Equals.'" *Journal of Medical Ethics* 29, no. 5 (2003): 307–312.

Glover, Jonathan. *Causing Death and Saving Lives*. New York: Penguin, 1977.

Goldstein, Joseph. "On Being Adult and Being an Adult in Secular Law." In *Adulthood*, edited by E. H. Erikson, 249–267. New York: W. W. Norton and Company, 1978.

Goyal, Madhav, Ravindra L. Mehta, Lawrence J. Schneiderman, and Ashwini R Sehgal. "Economic and Health Consequences of Selling a Kidney in India." *Journal of the American Medical Association* 288, no. 13 (2002): 1589–1593.

Grant, Ruth, and Jeremy Sugarman. "Ethics in Human Subjects Research: Do Incentives Matter?" *Journal of Medicine and Philosophy* 29, no. 6 (2004): 717–738.

Griffin, James. *Well-Being: Its Meaning, Measurement, and Moral Importance*. Oxford: Clarendon Press, 1986.

Gross, Hyman. "Privacy and Autonomy." In *Nomos XIII: Privacy*, edited by J. Roland Pennock and John W. Chapman, 169–181. New York: Atherton Press, 1971.

Hackler, Chris. *Health Care for an Aging Population*. Albany, NY: SUNY Press, 1994.

Haworth, Lawrence. "Dworkin on Autonomy." *Ethics* 102, no. 1 (1991): 129–139.

Heath, Joseph. "Liberal Autonomy and Consumer Sovereignty." In *Autonomy and the Challenges to Liberalism: New Essays*, edited by John Christman and Joel Anderson, 226–242. Cambridge: Cambridge University Press, 2005.

Hildt, Elisabeth. "Autonomy and Freedom of Choice in Prenatal Genetic Diagnosis." Medicine, *Health Care and Philosophy* 5, no. 1 (2002): 65–72.

Hill Jr., Thomas. "Servility and Self-Respect." In *Autonomy and Self-Respect*, edited by Thomas Hill, Jr., 4–18. Cambridge: Cambridge University Press, 1991.

———. *Dignity and Practical Reason in Kant's Moral Theory*. Ithaca, NY: Cornell University Press, 1992.

Hobbes, Thomas. *Leviathan*. London: Penguin Classics, 1982.

Holmberg, Scott, Steven Soloman, and Paul Blake. "Health and Economic Impacts of Anti-Microbial Resistance." *Reviews of Infectious Diseases* 9, no 6 (1987): 1065–1077.

Hughes, Paul M. "Ambivalence, Autonomy, and Organ Sales." *Southern Journal of Philosophy* 44, no. 2 (2006): 237–251.

———. "Exploitation, Autonomy, and the Case for Organ Sales." *International Journal of Applied Philosophy*, 12 no. 1 (1998): 89–95.

Hurka, Thomas. "Why Value Autonomy?" *Social Theory and Practice* 13, no. 3 (1987): 361–382.

Jackson, Jennifer. *Ethics in Medicine*. Cambridge: Polity Press, 2006.

Jones, James W. "Limits of Confidentiality: Disclosure of HIV Seropositivity." *Journal of Vascular Surgery* 38, no. 6 (2003): 1443–1444.

Kane, Robert. *Free Will and Values*. Albany, NY: State University of New York Press, 1985.

Kapitan, Tomis. "Autonomy and Manipulated Freedom." *Philosophical Perspectives* 14 (2000): 81–103.

Kershnar, Stephen. "A Liberal Case for Slavery." *Journal of Social Philosophy* 34, no. 4 (2003): 510–536.

Kohlberg, Lawrence. "Stage and Sequence: the Cognitive Development Approach to Socialization." In *The Handbook of Social Theory and Research*, edited by D. A. Goslin, 347–480. Chicago: Rand McNally, 1969.

Kristinsson, Sigurdur. "The Limits of Neutrality: Toward a Weakly Substantive Account of Autonomy." *Canadian Journal of Philosophy* 30, no. 2 (2000): 257–286.

Kupfer, Joseph. "Privacy, Autonomy, and Self-Concept." *American Philosophical Quarterly* 24, no. 1 (1987): 81–89.

Lehrer, Keith. *Metamind*. Oxford: Clarendon Press, 1990.

———. "Reason and Autonomy." In *Autonomy*, edited by Ellen Frankel Paul, Fred D. Miller Jr., Jeffrey Paul, 177–198. Cambridge: Cambridge University Press, 2003.

Levenbook, Barbara Baum. "Harming Someone After His Death." *Ethics* 94, no. 3 (1984): 407–419.

Levinsson, Henrik. "Autonomy and Metacognition—A Healthcare Perspective." PhD diss., Lund University, 2008.

Lippke, Richard. "Work, Privacy and Autonomy." *Public Affairs Quarterly* 3, no. 2 (1989): 41–55.

Lomasky, Loren. "Autonomy and Automobility." *The Independent Review* 2, no. 1 (1997): 5–28.

Lucas, J. L. *The Principles of Politics*. Oxford: Oxford University Press, 1966.

Luker, Kristin. *Taking Chances: Abortion and the Decision Not to Contracept*. Berkeley, CA: University of California Press, 1975.

Mason, Andrew. "Community and Autonomy: Logically Incompatible Values?" *Analysis* 51, no. 3 (1991): 160–166.

May, Thomas. *Bioethics in a Liberal Society*. Baltimore: The Johns Hopkins University Press, 2002.

McKenna, Michael. "The Relationship Between Autonomous and Morally Responsible Agency." In *Personal Autonomy: New Essays on Personal Autonomy and Its Role in Contemporary Moral Philosophy*, edited by James Stacey Taylor, 205–234. Cambridge: Cambridge University Press, 2005.

McLeod, Carolyn. *Self-Trust and Reproductive Autonomy*. Cambridge: MIT Press, 2002.

Mele, Alfred R. *Autonomous Agents: From Self-Control to Autonomy*. New York: Oxford University Press, 1995.

———. "History and Personal Autonomy." *Canadian Journal of Philosophy* 23, no. 2 (1993): 271–280.

Merry, Alan, and Alexander McCall Smith. *Errors, Medicine and the Law*. Cambridge: Cambridge University Press, 2001.

Meyers, Diana Tietjens. "Feminism and Womens' Autonomy: The Challenge of Female Genital Cutting." *Metaphilosophy* 31, no. 5 (2000): 469–491.

———. "Intersectional Identity and the Authentic Self? Opposites Attract!" In *Relational Autonomy: Feminist Perspectives on Autonomy, Agency, and the Social Self*, edited by Catriona Mackenzie and Natalie Stoljar, 151–180. Oxford: Oxford University Press, 2000.

———. *Self, Society, and Personal Choice*. New York: Columbia University Press, 1991.

Meyerson, Denise. "When Are My Actions Due to Me?" *Analysis* 54, no. 3 (1994): 171–174.

Michalowski, Sabine. *Medical Confidentiality and Crime*. Aldershot, England: Ashgate Publishing, 2003.

Mill, J. S. *On Liberty*. Edited by Elizabeth Rapaport. Indianapolis: Hackett Publishing Company, Inc., 1978.

Miller, Bruce. "Autonomy and the Refusal of Lifesaving Treatment." *Hastings Center Report* 11, no. 4 (1981): 22–28.

Mills, Claudia. "Choice and Circumstance." *Ethics* 109, no. 1 (1998): 154–165.

Milton, John. *Paradise Lost*. London: Penguin Classics, 2000.

Nagel, Thomas. "Death." In *The Metaphysics of Death*, edited by John Martin Fischer, 59–69. Stanford, CA: Stanford University Press, 1993.

Noggle, Robert. "Autonomy and the Paradox of Self-Creation: Infinite Regresses, Finite Selves, and the Limits of Authenticity." In *Personal Autonomy: New Essays on Personal Autonomy and Its Role in Contemporary Moral Philosophy*, edited by James Stacey Taylor, 87–108. Cambridge: Cambridge University Press, 2005.

———. "Autonomy, Value, and Conditioned Desire." *American Philosophical Quarterly* 32, no. 1 (1995): 57–69.

———. "Kantian Respect and Particular Persons." *Canadian Journal of Philosophy* 26, no. 3 (1999): 449–477.

———. "The Public Conception of Autonomy and Critical Self-Reflection." *Southern Journal of Philosophy* 35, no. 4 (1997): 495–515.

Nozick, Robert. *Anarchy, State, and Utopia*. Oxford: Blackwell, 1974.

Oshana, Marina A. L. *Personal Autonomy in Society*. Aldershot, England: Ashgate Publishing, 2006.

———. "The Misguided Marriage of Responsibility and Autonomy." *The Journal of Ethics* 6, no. 3 (2002): 261–280.

———. "Wanton Responsibility." *The Journal of Ethics* 2, no. 1 (1998): 261–276.

Parent, William A. "Recent Work on the Concept of Privacy." *American Philosophical Quarterly* 20, no. 4 (1983): 341–355.

Pears, David. *Motivated Irrationality*. Oxford: Clarendon Press, 1984.

Peters, R. S. "Freedom and the Development of the Free Man." In *Educational Judgments: Papers in the Philosophy of Education*, edited by James F. Doyle, 119–142. London: Routledge, 1973.

Piaget, Jean. *The Moral Judgment of the Child*. New York: Basic Books, 1966.

Pitcher, George. "The Misfortunes of the Dead." In *The Metaphysics of Death*, edited by John Martin Fischer, 157–168. Stanford, CA: Stanford University Press, 1993.

Polsby, Daniel D. "Regulation of Foods and Drugs and Libertarian Ideals: Perspectives of a Fellow-Traveller." In *Problems of Market Liberalism*, edited by Ellen Frankel Paul, Fred D. Miller Jr., Jeffrey Paul, 209–242. Cambridge: Cambridge University Press, 1998.

Portmore, Douglas. "Desire Fulfillment and Posthumous Harm." *American Philosophical Quarterly* 44, no. 1 (2007): 27–38.

Rachels, James. "Why Privacy Is Important." *Philosophy and Public Affairs* 4, no. 4 (1975): 323–33.

Rawls, John. "Kantian Constructivism in Moral Theory." *The Journal of Philosophy* 77, no. 9 (1980): 554–572.

Raz, Joseph. *The Morality of Freedom.* Oxford: Oxford University Press, 1986.

Richardson, Henry. "Autonomy's Many Normative Presuppositions." *American Philosophical Quarterly* 38, no. 3 (1991): 287–303.

Rosenbaum, Stephen. "Epicurus and Annihilation." *The Philosophical Quarterly* 39, no. 154 (1989): 81–90.

Ross, W. D. *Foundations of Ethics.* Oxford: Clarendon Press, 1939.

Rovane, Carol. *The Bounds of Agency.* Princeton, NJ: Princeton University Press, 2007.

Santiago, John. "Personal Autonomy: What's Content Got to Do with It?" *Social Theory and Practice* 31, no. 1 (2005): 77–104.

Scanlon, Thomas. "A Theory of Freedom of Expression." *Philosophy and Public Affairs* 1, no. 2 (1972): 204–226.

Scarre, Geoffrey. "Archaeology and Respect for the Dead." *Journal of Applied Philosophy* 20, no. 3 (2003): 237–249.

Schier, Flint. "The Kantian Gulag: Autonomy and the Liberal Conception of Freedom." In *Virtue and Taste: Essays on Politics, Ethics, and Aesthetics in Memory of Flint Schier,* edited by Dudley Knowles and John Skorupski, 1–17. Oxford: Blackwell, 1993.

Schneider, Carl E. *The Practice of Autonomy: Patients, Doctors, and Medical Decisions.* New York: Oxford University Press, 1998.

Schroder, Timothy, and Nomy Arpaly. "Alienation and Externality." *Canadian Journal of Philosophy* 29, no. 3 (1999): 371–388.

Schwartz, Lisa, Paul Preece, and Ron Hendry. *Medical Ethics: A Case-Based Approach.* Oxford: Saunders Ltd, 2002.

Sells, R. A. "Voluntarism of Consent." In *Organ Replacement Therapy: Ethics, Justice, Commerce,* edited by W. Land and J. Dossestor, 18–24. New York: Springer-Verlag, 1991.

Shakespeare, William. *Othello.* Edited by Edward Pechter. New York: W. W. Norton and Company, 2003.

Sher, George. *Beyond Neutrality: Perfectionism and Politics.* Cambridge: Cambridge University Press, 1997.

Shoemaker, David. "Caring, Identification, and Agency." *Ethics* 114, no. 1 (2003): 88–118.

Smith, Angela M. "Identification and Responsibility." In *Moral Responsibility and Ontology,* edited by Ton van den Beld, 233–246. Dordrecht: Kluwer Academic Publishers, 2000.

Smith, Janet. "The Pre-eminence of Autonomy in Bioethics." In *Human Lives: Critical Essays on Consequentialist Bioethics,* edited by D. S. Oderberg and J. A. Laing, 182–195. London/New York: Macmillan/St. Martin's Press, 1997.

Spriggs, Merle. "Can We Help Addicts Become More Autonomous? Inside the Mind of an Addict." *Bioethics* 17, nos. 5–6 (2003): 542–554.

Stein, Gertrude. *Everybody's Autobiography.* New York: Cooper Square Publishers, 1971.

Stoljar, Natalie. "Autonomy and the Feminist Intuition." In *Relational Autonomy: Feminist Perspectives on Autonomy, Agency, and the Social Self,* edited by Catriona Mackenzie and Natalie Stoljar, 94–111. Oxford: Oxford University Press, 2000.

Stone, Carolyn M. "Autonomy, Emotions, and Desires: Some Problems Concerning R. F. Dearden's Account of Autonomy." *Journal of Philosophy of Education* 24, no. 2 (1990): 271–283.

Sturgeon, Theodore. "The Dark Room." In *The Golden Helix,* edited by Theodore Sturgeon, 191–227. Garden City, NY: Nelson Doubleday, 1979.

Tausk, Victor. "On the Origin of the 'Influencing Machine' in Schizophrenia." *Psychoanalytic Quarterly* 2 (1933): 519–556.

Taylor, James Stacey. "Autonomy and Informed Consent: A Much Misunderstood Relationship." *Journal of Value Inquiry* 38, no. 3 (2004): 383–391.

———. "Autonomy and Informed Consent on the Navajo Reservation." *Journal of Social Philosophy* 35, no. 4 (2004): 506–516.

———. "Autonomy and Political Liberalism." *Social Theory and Practice* 32, no. 3 (2006): 497–510.

———. "Autonomy, Duress, and Coercion." *Social Philosophy & Policy* 20, no. 2 (2003): 127–155.

———. "Autonomy, Inducements, and Organ Sales." In *Philosophical Reflections on Medical Ethics*, edited by Nafsika Athanassoulis, 135–159. London: Palgrave Macmillan, 2005.

———. "Identification and Quasi-Desires." *Philosophical Papers* 34, no. 1 (2005): 111–136.

———. "Introduction." In *Personal Autonomy: New Essays on Personal Autonomy and Its Role in Contemporary Moral Philosophy*, edited by James Stacey Taylor, 1–29. Cambridge: Cambridge University Press, 2005.

———. "Plea Bargains, Constraining Options, and Respect for Autonomy." *Public Affairs Quarterly* 18, no. 3 (2004): 249–264.

———. "Review of *Necessity, Volition, and Love*." *Philosophical Quarterly* 51, no. 202 (2001): 114–116.

———. *Stakes and Kidneys: Why Markets in Human Body Parts are Morally Imperative*. Aldershot, England: Ashgate Publishing, 2005.

———. "The Myth of Posthumous Harm." *American Philosophical Quarterly* 42, no. 4 (2005): 311–322.

———. "Willing Addicts, Unwilling Addicts, and Acting of One's Own Free Will." *Philosophia* 33, nos. 1–4 (2005): 237–262.

Thalberg, Irving. "Hierarchical Analyses of Unfree Action." In *The Inner Citadel: Essays on Individual Autonomy*, edited by John Christman, 123–136. New York: Oxford University Press, 1989.

———. "Socialization and Autonomous Behavior." *Tulane Studies in Philosophy* 28 (1979): 21–37.

Thomson, Judith Jarvis. "The Right to Privacy." In *Philosophical Dimensions of Privacy: An Anthology*, edited by Ferdinand D. Schoeman, 272–289. Cambridge: Cambridge University Press, 1984.

Titmuss, Richard. *The Gift Relationship: From Human Blood to Social Policy*. Edited by Ann Oakley and John Ashton. New York: The New Press, 1997.

Tollefsen, Christopher. "*Sic Et Non*: Some Disputed Questions in Reproductive Ethics." In *Handbook of Bioethics: Taking Stock of the Field from a Philosophical Perspective*, edited by George Khushf, 381–414. Dordrecht: Springer, 2004.

Tunick, Mark. "Does Privacy Undermine Community?" *Journal of Value Inquiry* 35, no. 4 (2001): 529–531.

Varelius, Jukka. "On Taylor on Autonomy and Informed Consent." *Journal of Value Inquiry* 40, no 4 (2006): 451–459.

Vargas, Manuel. "Review of *Personal Autonomy: New Essays on Personal Autonomy and Its Role in Contemporary Moral Philosophy*," edited by James Stacey Taylor. *Notre Dame Philosophical Reviews* (15th August 2006). Online at: http://ndpr.nd.edu/review.cfm?id=7363. Last accessed October 14th, 2008.

Velleman, J. David. "Identification and Identity." In *Contours of Agency: Essays on Themes from Harry Frankfurt*, edited by Sarah Buss and Lee Overton, 91–123. Cambridge: MIT Press, 2002.

———. "What Happens When Someone Acts?" *Mind* 101, no. 403 (1992): 461–481.

Waller, Bruce. *The Natural Selection of Autonomy*. Albany, NY: The State University of New York Press, 1998.

Warren, Samuel D., and Louis D. Brandeis. "The Right to Privacy [the Implicit Made Explicit]." in *Philosophical Dimensions of Privacy: An Anthology*, edited by Ferdinand D. Schoeman, 75–103. Cambridge: Cambridge University Press, 1984.

Watson, Gary. "Free Agency." In *The Inner Citadel: Essays on Individual Autonomy*, edited by John Christman, 109–122. New York: Oxford University Press, 1989.

———. "Volitional Necessities." In *Contours of Agency: Essays on Themes from Harry Frankfurt*, edited by Sarah Buss and Lee Overton, 129–159. Cambridge: MIT Press, 2002.

Waugh, Evelyn. *Decline and Fall*. London: Chapman Hall, 1974.

Wertheimer, Alan. *Coercion*. Princeton, NJ: Princeton University Press, 1987.

Westin, Alan. "The Origins of Modern Claims to Privacy." In *Philosophical Dimensions of Privacy: An Anthology*, edited by Ferdinand D. Schoeman, 56–74. Cambridge: Cambridge University Press, 1984.

White, Amy E. "The Morality of an Internet Market in Human Ova." *Journal of Value Inquiry* 40, nos. 2–3 (2006): 311–321.

Williams, Bernard. "A Critique of Utilitarianism." In *Utilitarianism: For and Against*, edited by J. J. C. Smart and Bernard Williams, 77–150. Cambridge: Cambridge University Press, 1973.

———. "Moral Incapacity." In *Making Sense of Humanity and Other Philosophical Papers 1982–1993*, edited by Bernard Williams, 46–55. Cambridge: Cambridge University Press, 1995.

Wilson, James. "Is Respect for Autonomy Defensible?" *Journal of Medical Ethics* 33, no. 6 (2007): 353–356.

Winnicott, D. W. "Ego Distortion in Terms of True and False Self." In *The Maturational Processes and the Facilitating Environment*, edited by D. W. Winnicott, 140–152. London: Hogarth Press, 1965.

Wolff, R. P. *In Defense of Anarchism*. New York: Harper and Row, 1970.

Woodward, B. "Confidentiality, Consent and Autonomy in the Physician–Patient Relationship." *Health Care Analysis* 9, no. 3 (2001): 337–351.

Yeide Jr., Harry. "The Many Faces of Autonomy." *Journal of Clinical Ethics* 3, no. 4 (1992): 269–274.

Young, Robert. *Personal Autonomy: Beyond Negative and Positive Liberty*. London: Croom Helm Ltd, 1986.

———. "The Value of Autonomy." *The Philosophical Quarterly* 32, no. 126 (1982): 35–44.

Zutlevics, T. L. "Markets and the Needy: Organ Sales or Aid?" *Journal of Applied Philosophy* 18, no. 3 (2001): 297–302.

# Index

**A**

*Ab Initio* Problem, 51, 53–55, 105, 106, 107, 108
abortion, 154
addict, willing, 58–59
addict, unwilling, 15, 58–59
addiction, 3, 15, 40, 58, 172n15
agential desires, 43, 44, 59, 70, 164n38, 172n23, 176n33, 190n25
alienation, 12, 46, 56, 58, 61, 75, 176n28
ambivalence, 3, 83, 89, 91–93
Amish, 158
antibiotics, 87–88, 183n24
Appelbaum, S., 130
applied ethics, 16, 18, 45–47, 173n33
Arpaly, Nomy, 19, 20, 22, 23–35, 45–47, 167n19, 168n22, 168n24, 169n30, 169n32, 169n39, 170n42, 170n43, 170n51, 173n30, 173n33, 173n34, 174n36, 182n11, 188–189n4
autonomy: as absence of external causation, 19, 22; as agent-autonomy (*see* identification); ahistorical accounts of, 164n45; as authenticity, 20, 30–33, 35; as authority over personal choices, 19, 22; as bare agency, 19, 22; as capacity, 19, 21, 24, 25, 34; as character type, 19, 21; as competence for medical decision-making, 19, 22; as condition, 19, 21; as critical reflection, 19, 22; as dignity, 19, 22; failure to respect, 27, 28, 30, 115–116, 136; as identification. *See* identification;

content-neutral, xv, 17, 63–66, 66–70, 71–77, 77–80, 81; for which external restrictions are irrelevant, 20, 22; externalist; xiv, 15–17, 62, 157; as freedom from control or restriction on choice, 19, 20, 22; as freedom of the will (*see* freedom of the will); as heroic, 20, 34, 35; historical account of, 12–13, 13–15, 17; as independence, 19, 22; as independence of mind, 20, 26, 35; as individuality, 19, 22; instrumental value of, xvi, 6, 15, 25, 27, 84–85, 86, 92, 108, 111, 112, 129, 139–140, 141, 142, 144, 154, 155, 156, 193n1, 193n2, 193n29; interpersonal comparisons of, 155; intrinsic value of, xvi, 84, 85, 86, 92–93, 112, 140, 142–144, 144–154, 155, 158, 195n25; as knowledge of our own interests, 19, 22; as morally responsible agency, 19, 22; as negative liberty, 19, 21; as normative moral autonomy 20, 26–30, 35; normative competence account of, 65, 70, 80–81; as ownership-taking, 19, 22; as personal efficacy, 20, 24–26, 35; as a political concept, 16, 17, 38, 49, 107, 157; as a political designation, 19; practical, xiii, xiv, 4, 6–17, 18, 35, 51, 63, 64–66, 78–79, 80, 81, 84, 106, 107, 116, 123, 131, 135, 139–140; as positive liberty, 19, 21; as relation to the world, 19, 22; as reasons-responsiveness, 20, 34–35;

as responsibility, 19, 22; as a right, 19, 22; as rule-governed activity, 19, 22; as self-assertion, 19, 22; as self-control, 19, 22; as self-governed agency, 19, 22; as self-identification, 20, 33–34, 35; as self-knowledge, 19, 22; as self-rule, 19, 21–22, 39; substantive, xv, 17, 65, 67, 69, 70–77, 77–80, 81, 82, 177n2; violation of, 26, 27, 115–116, 154

**B**

backwards causation, 150–152
Beauchamp, T. L., xiii, 130, 134
Berkeley, George, 147–148
Benn, Stanley I., 119, 119–120, 121, 127
Benson, Paul, 47, 77–79, 177n2
Berlin, Isaiah, 19, 21
Berofsky, Bernard, 107, 169n32
Big Brother, 119
bioethics, xiii, xiv, xv, 1, 2, 4, 17, 18, 19, 22, 25, 34, 36, 37, 38, 49, 50, 51, 62,77, 82, 84, 96, 108, 112, 114, 124, 127, 129, 130, 140, 157, 158, 173n34; and content-neutral autonomy, 63–66; importance of autonomy for, 45–47; value of autonomy in, 141–156
bioethical public policy, 154–155
Biological constraints, 109
Bixby, Jerome, 25
Brandeis, Louis B., 114
Bratman, Michael, 23, 176n28
Buchanan, Allen, 110–111
Buss, Sarah, 162n20

**C**

Callahan, Joan, 152–153
*Canturbury v. Spence*, 130
Cherry, Mark J., 109
Childress, James F., 130, 134
Christian morality, xiii, 177n3
Christman, John, xiii, 12–13, 21, 53–55, 66, 67–70, 105–106, 172n12, 174–175n1, 178n8, 179n29, 186n30
*Cobbs v. Grant*, 133
coercion, 3, 40, 45, 136, 139, 154
commercial surrogate pregnancy. *See* surrogate pregnancy
commitment, xv, 17, 57, 82, 97, 110–112

commitments. *See* core desires
community, 110, 111
compatibilism, 54
Complex Autonomy Theories, 45–47
constraint, xvi, 63, 66, 69, 82, 95, 96–113, 158, 166n16, 177n2, 178n25, 180n50, 185n1, 185n8, 188n50
constraining options, 83, 84, 85–88, 88–89, 110
contingent preferences, 104–107
control, 4–6, 7, 16, 20, 26, 34, 41, 52, 54, 68–70, 73, 75, 78, 100, 101, 102, 105, 120–127, 128, 131, 132–133, 136–137
core desires, 123
cosmetic surgery, 12, 25, 83, 84, 111
Cuypers, Stefaan, 105, 106, 186n30

**D**

deception, 3–6, 29, 45, 130–131, 136, 139, 148, 149, 170n43, 172n24, 178–179n25, 191n8, 195n25
Dennett, Daniel C., 122–123
Dickens, Charles, 71, 174n42
Double, Richard, 72, 163n28
duress, 127, 136, 139, 191n29
Dworkin, Gerald, xiv, 19, 20, 21–22, 35, 38–39, 42, 66, 67–70, 79, 93, 153, 161n8, 166n12, 166–167n16, 178n25, 181n2, 184n35
Dwyer, Susan J., 1

**E**

Economic constraints, 107–109, 155, 187n37, 187n42
elective amputation, 83
Elster, Jon, 67, 68–70, 71–72, 73, 74
Engelhardt, H. Tristram Jr., xiii, 1, 185n8
epidemiological research, 128
epistemological problems, 16, 176n22
eudaimoistic life, 141
experience machine, the, 146, 147–148
extreme voluntarism, 96, 98–102, 103, 105, 107, 134

**F**

Faden, R.R., 130
fast action, 34–35
Feinberg, Joel, 19, 35, 146–147, 149–153
feminist intuition, 77–80, 180n48

Fowles, John 28
Frankfurt, Harry G., xiii, 9, 10,
 20–21, 23, 30–33, 35, 37–39,
 47–48, 51, 52–55, 57–59, 60,
 97, 102–105, 161n6, 168n23,
 176n28, 186n16
free will, xiv, 10, 39, 41, 43, 52
freedom of the will, 19, 21, 37, 52, 54
Fried, Charles, 116
Friedman, Marilyn, 105, 142, 186n30

**G**

Gertrude Stein Problem, the, 1, 18,
 165n1
Gilligan, Carol, 169n32
Griffin, James, 194n4
Gross, Hyman P., 116

**H**

Hackler, Chris, 117
hedonistic assumption, the 146–154
Hendry, Ron, 116–117
heteronomy, 9, 12, 66–69, 164n38
heteronomous. *See* heteronomy
hierarchical analyses, 39–40
Hill, Thomas E., Jr., 26, 80
Hughes, Paul M., 3, 85–86
human research subjects, 91, 94, 96
Hurka, Thomas, 142–144, 154,
 196n48

**I**

identification, xiv, xv, 10, 17, 20,
 23–24, 29, 30, 33, 35, 36,
 37–50, 51–62, 63, 157, 162n22,
 176n33; attitudinal account of,
 56; as internalist concept, 61–62;
 structural account of, 56–57
Incompleteness Problem, the. *See*
 Regress-cum-Incompleteness
 Problem, the
informed consent, xv, xv1, 17, 37,
 129, 130–140, 141, 155, 158,
 191–192n12
irresistible offers, 83, 89–91

**J**

Jones, James W., 114

**K**

Kant, Immanuel, xiii, 30, 48, 103
kidney sales. *See*, markets in human
 organs.
Kierkegaard, Soren, 76

Kristinsson, Sigurdur, 64, 66–70, 81,
 177n2
Kupfer, Joseph, 118–119, 119–120,
 121, 127, 189–190n16

**L**

Lehrer, Keith, 23
Levenbook, Barbara Baum, 152–153
Lidz, C.W., 130
Lomasky, Loren, 168–169n27,
 183n24
Luker, Kristin, 77
Luther, Martin, 31, 102–103

**M**

markets in human organs, xiv, 83,
 85–86, 90, 91, 94, 95, 96, 113,
 83, 139, 155, 158
markets in human ova, 83
manipulation, 3–6, 13, 16, 33, 41–42,
 45, 51, 53, 54, 55, 60–61, 72,
 130–131, 136, 139, 144–154,
 162n16, 163n23, 163n24
May, Thomas, 131
McKenna, Michael, 162n16
medical confidentiality. *See* patient
 confidentiality
Meisel, A., 130
Mele, Alfred, 4–6
Meyers, Diana, 77–78
Michalowski, Sabine, 114
Mills, Claudia, 143–144
Milton, John, 80–81
moral incapacity. *See* unthinkability
morning-after pill, 177n5

**N**

Navajo, 158
negligence, 131, 132–233, 135, 136,
 138, 139, 140
neo-existentialism. *See* extreme voluntarism
Noggle, Robert, 23, 168n23
nonalienation, 12, 164n40
Nozick, Robert, 145–146, 153

**O**

Occam's Razor, 14
options, xv, 15, 63, 66, 67, 68, 83,
 84, 85–88, 88–89, 90, 91–93,
 93–94, 95, 103, 104, 105, 108,
 109, 110, 113, 131, 132, 142–
 144, 153–155, 158, 168n27,
 182n11, 182n12, 182–183n19,

184n28, 184n35, 188–189n4, 196n48
Orwell, George, 119
Oshana, Marina A.L., 79, 187n37
*Othello*. See Othello
Othello, 4–5, 13, 15, 16, 33, 41–42, 62, 75–76, 125, 132, 134, 144–145, 147, 148–149, 151, 153, 194n17

**P**

patient confidentiality, xvi, 114, 115, 116, 128–129, 130, 141, 155, 158
patient-physician relation, the 154
Pears, David, 61
personal identity, 48, 56–57, 106–107, 175n21, 176n22
Piaget, Jean, 118
Pitcher, George, 150–153
posthumous harm, 145–153
poverty. *See* economic constraints
Preece, Paul, 116–117
preference structure, 53–55, 81, 98–102, 103, 105, 106, 107, 111, 175n11, 185n4
prenatal genetic diagnosis, 83
prescription drugs, 136, 154
privacy, xv, 17, 114–129, 130
Problem of Authority, the. See *Ab Initio* Problem, the.
Problem of Manipulation, the, 13, 51, 53, 54–55, 60, 175n11
public health, 154

**R**

Rachels, James, 127, 190n22
radical freedom, 97–98. *See also* extreme voluntarism
Raz, Joseph, 108, 182n12
Regress Problem, the. *See* Regress-cum-Incompleteness Problem, the
Regress-cum-Incompleteness Problem, the, 52, 53, 54–55, 57–58
reproductive technology, 37
Requirement of Universal Endorsement, the, 10
Richardson, Henry, 71–77, 80, 179n32, 180n43
Ross, W.D., 146

**S**

Santiago, John, 80, 179n31
satisfaction, 8–9, 10–11, 12, 13, 15

Schwartz, Lisa, 116–117
Schier, Flint, 180n50
scopolamine, 84
self-control, 4, 19, 23, 32, 34
self-deception, 13, 67, 71–73
self-identity, 101
self-reflection, 12–13
sex change, 111
Smith, Janet, 154
Soviet gulags, 93–94
surrogate pregnancy, 83
surveillance, 120, 120–121, 122, 124, 125, 145
sterilization, 111
Stoljar, Natalie, 77–80, 180n48
Stone, Carolyn M., 110, 111
Sturgeon, Theodore, 104–105

**T**

Tausk, Victor, 118
Taylor, James Stacey, 19, 174n39, 174–175n1
temptation, 83, 89, 91=93, 184n34, 188n50
Thalberg, Irving, 172n14, 180n48
Thomson, Judith Jarvis, 117, 122–123
Titmuss, Richard, 182–183n19
Type A situations, 165n51, 182n12

**U**

unthinkability, 31, 32, 33, 102–105, 184n30, 186n16

**V**

Varelius, Jukka, 131, 136–139, 192n20, 193n25, 193n26, 103n27, 103n28, 193n30
Vargas, Manuel, 19, 22–23, 35
Velleman, David J., 13–15, 23, 30–32, 59–60, 168n23, 170n52, 170–171n53
volitional necessity, 31, 32, 33, 102–105, 186n16

**W**

wanton, 2, 8, 9–10, 21, 26, 104, 163n35, 175n20
Warren, Samuel D., 114
Watson, Gary, 23, 53, 57, 168n23
Waugh, Evelyn, 9
weakness of will, 40, 93
well-being, 15, 84, 141, 149, 150–152, 191n10, 192n14, 193n27, 193–194n2

will, 9, 10, 19, 21, 30, 31, 32, 33,
   37–50, 51–62, 85, 87, 90,
   93, 94, 97, 98, 99, 102, 103,
   104, 168n23, 171n4, 171n6,
   174n37, 174n39, 174n41;
   constitutive, 98, 102, 103, 104,
   185n5, 186n16; Hobbesian, 99,
   172n9, 175n6, 185n3, 185n5;
   substantial (*see* constitutive)

Williams, Bernard, 123
Winnicutt, D.W., 31–32

**Y**
Yeide, Harry Jr., 1

**Z**
Zutlevics, T.L., 87
zombie drug. *See* scopolamine

T - #0174 - 071024 - C0 - 229/152/12 - PB - 9780415890564 - Gloss Lamination